Hysterectomy for Benign Conditions

Hysterectomy for Benign Conditions

Sun Kuie Tay

MBBS (London), MD (London), FRCOG

Clinical Professor and Senior Consultant Obstetrician & Gynecologist

Singapore General Hospital, Singapore &
Duke-NUS Medical School, Singapore

World Scientific

NEW JERSEY · LONDON · SINGAPORE · BEIJING · SHANGHAI · HONG KONG · TAIPEI · CHENNAI · TOKYO

Published by

World Scientific Publishing Co. Pte. Ltd.

5 Toh Tuck Link, Singapore 596224

USA office: 27 Warren Street, Suite 401-402, Hackensack, NJ 07601

UK office: 57 Shelton Street, Covent Garden, London WC2H 9HE

British Library Cataloguing-in-Publication Data

A catalogue record for this book is available from the British Library.

HYSTERECTOMY FOR BENIGN CONDITIONS

ISBN 978-981-124-392-9 (hardcover)
ISBN 978-981-124-570-1 (paperback)
ISBN 978-981-124-393-6 (ebook for institutions)
ISBN 978-981-124-394-3 (ebook for individuals)

For any available supplementary material, please visit
https://www.worldscientific.com/worldscibooks/10.1142/12474#t=suppl

Printed in Singapore

Contents

Preface

I started my career in obstetrics and gynecology on August 1, 1982 when I was taken in as a greenhorn senior house officer in London's Royal Northern Hospital, the home ground of the late great surgeon teachers Mr Hamilton Bailey and Mr McNeill Love. On the first day, Mr Michael Pugh, a senior consultant obstetrician and gynecologist, said to me: "You are given this training position because you are totally new in gynecology. We can teach you properly before you develop any bad habits in gynecology. We will make sure that you will be a confident and competent gynecologist. You must help women!" These words still echo vividly in my mind.

From many ingenious, generous, and inspiring teachers I have learned both simple and sophisticated surgical skills while witnessing the practice of wisdom in the untiring dedication of good doctors. Together with a process of lifelong, continual learning and research, the unique experience of active patient care has given me a fulfilling and satisfying professional career in gynecology.

The three phases of my gynecologic career include my specialty training years in the United Kingdom from 1982 to 1987, the professional consolidation years from 1988 to 1996 at Singapore General Hospital, and my senior faculty years at the same institution from 1997 till today. A review of surgical logbooks between 1997 and 2017 reveals the registration of more than ten thousand surgical cases I had performed personally. Among these were 2,939 cases of laparotomy, 1,445 cases of laparoscopy, and 342 cases of vaginal hysterectomy (see Appendix). For this book, I have chosen hysterectomy as the procedure to share some aspects of my knowledge and skills in gynecologic surgery with gynecologists and surgeons both in training and in practice. Hysterectomy is not only the most common major surgery in women; it also encompasses the entire theory and principle of all surgeries. It involves surgical approaches through traditional open abdominal surgery, the less invasive laparoscopic techniques, and surgery through the natural passage of the vagina, which is genuinely the most minimally invasive surgery.

The first principle that all surgical students have to remember is that surgery is nothing but a controlled assault to a human body. It is the power of nature that heals the wound. A good surgery inflicts a wound that causes the least violation to the principle of healing by nature. Residents learning to do hysterectomy should, therefore, appreciate that it is far more important to do one case correctly than to do ten cases but repeat the same mistake ten times.

The second principle of surgery that I uphold vigorously is the avoidance of curing a patient's disease by surgery only to let him or her suffer another problem from complications of the surgery. Continual modification of surgical techniques and innovation are central to a surgeon's daily activity. There may be incremental improvements by evolution or by innovative changes in a leapfrog revolution. Each new generation of gynecologists should aspire and determine to do hysterectomy better than surgeons of past years. This second principle of surgery is based on a sound foundation of the first principle.

This is a book of the first principle of surgery, not a mere manual of steps of hysterectomy. It emphasizes the core surgical expertise of a gynecologic surgeon who plays a central role in shaping the female patient's experience and outcome in the journey of hysterectomy. It is written with the objective of providing residents a sound understanding of the principle of hysterectomy based on knowledge of anatomy and physiology. It forms a basis for residents to adapt techniques for hysterectomy according to circumstances of pathology, pelvic environment, and his or her surgical dexterity, thereby exercising the second principle of surgery. In essence, the foundation of a successful surgery is built on attributes known as the three "As": Anatomy, Access, and Ability.

Total abdominal hysterectomy for benign conditions is the anatomical, physiological, and surgical basis of all ramifications of different types of hysterectomy. This is the procedure for which I will provide specific details. The relevant technical approaches for laparoscopic and vaginal hysterectomy are sufficiently described so that residents can achieve practical competency.

While it is not my intention to provide a comprehensive critical review of the merits and demerits of various methods or techniques for hysterectomy, I illustrate in this book the surgical principle and rationale that guide my own practice of hysterectomy for benign conditions, with full cognizance of the universally acknowledged truth that a surgical procedure is right only when the right surgeon operates on the right patient for the right disease.

I cannot further emphasize the significance of meticulous preparation and care for patients during the peri-operative period. A comprehensive chapter on this aspect is included in this book to highlight relevant measures for optimization of the patient's physiology and anatomy and for prevention, early recognition, and appropriate management of complications and injuries specific to hysterectomy. Peri-operative care forms a part of the integral philosophy of surgery, of which hysterectomy is but one.

Tay Sun Kuie MD, FRCOG
Singapore 2021

Foreword

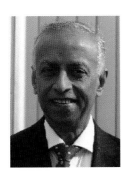

Sir Sabaratnam Arulkumaran
PhD DSc FRCS FRCOG
Professor Emeritus of Obstetrics & Gynaecology

Hysterectomy for Benign Conditions

by Professor Tay Sun Kuie

I was delighted to read this "surgical classic" of *Hysterectomy for Benign Conditions* by Professor Tay Sun Kuie, which encompasses the principles and practice of surgery and comprehensive care that includes the different dimensions of commitment, compassion, communication, competence, confidence, and team care. Every chapter is well written and adheres to the basic principles of patient-centered care, anatomy, physiology, and pathology. It is clear that this book has been authored by an experienced surgeon who has performed more than 10,000 surgical laparotomy operations. All the chapters are well illustrated with clear and colorful photographs that complement the description in the text. The book opens with a discussion of the "what" and "why" of hysterectomy — describing the meaning of hysterectomy and dealing with the issues of "pro-hysterectomy", which involves the indications for the procedure, "anti-hysterectomy" which discusses possible alternatives, and "consequences of hysterectomy" which deals with resolution of pathology and possible complications. This chapter reminds the reader of the Hippocratic oath, the principle of "primum non nocera" (do no harm), and the ethical tenet that the well-being of patients should be of primary interest.

The second chapter deals with the initial step of laparotomy for hysterectomy, describing in detail the midline and the different types of transverse incisions, the original and the modifications. Meticulous care is given to describe anatomical landmarks and the layer-by-layer opening and closure of the abdomen, possible difficulties, and how to overcome them. The section on principles guiding the selection of the type of abdominal incision has useful advice for any practising surgeon. The third chapter deals with the anatomy of pelvic structures relevant to hysterectomy. The detailed description of the uterus is followed by description of fasciae, folds, and ligaments with colored real-time surgical pictures, which help to identify the structures. Brief descriptions of blood supply, nerve supply, lymphatic drainage, and pelvic floor muscles are provided, which are useful in guiding the execution of clean surgery and avoiding accidental injury. The fourth chapter deals with the procedure of total and subtotal abdominal hysterectomy with and without bilateral salpingo-oopherectomy (BSO). It deals with the preparation of the bladder, skin, and instruments required followed by laparotomy as described in the previous chapter. It then deals with the meticulous surgery based on the anatomical description of each structure that connects the uterus to the lateral pelvic wall, adjacent structures, and the vagina vault. Descriptions are complimented by color photographs every step of the way for easy understanding. Moreover, the importance of confirmation haemostasis and the pelvic drainage tube is emphasized. The fifth chapter is dedicated to vaginal hysterectomy (VH). A brief discussion of the advantages of VH over AH is followed by indications and contraindications for VH. A description of the technique of VH begins with intraoperative preparation followed by a discussion of the handling of each pedicle and closure of the peritoneal cavity and the vaginal vault. Modifications to VH such as salpingectomy, VH with BSO, VH of large volume uterus, and laparoscopically assisted VH are also described.

Chapter 6 deals with laparoscopy for hysterectomy. It starts with the development of laparoscopy, its early era, and the uniqueness of laparoscopy, describing surgical skill development and adaptation, maintenance of sustained pneumoperitoneum, ergonomics of laparoscopic surgery, and surgical complications. Surgical pelvic anatomy for laparoscopy, especially the vascularity of the abdominal wall and that posterior to the abdominal peritoneum, is described, which helps in avoiding vascular injuries. Applied physiology for laparoscopy, contraindications, risk factors for conversion to laparotomy, and risks with postsurgical adhesions are described. Chapter 7 begins its description of the laparoscopic hysterectomy (LH) procedure with the classification as laparoscopy-assisted vaginal hysterectomy (LAVH), laparoscopic hysterectomy, total laparoscopic hysterectomy, and laparoscopic supracervical hysterectomy. This is followed by a comparison between LH, VH, and AH. Indications and contraindications of LH are discussed. Step-by-step descriptions of different methods of creating pneumoperitoneum followed by careful surgery through identifying each pedicle, achieving haemostasis, removing the uterus, and closing the vaginal vault are described in detail with photographic illustrations included. Chapter 8 deals with perioperative care, starting with pre-operative care to review the decision for hysterectomy, the pre-operative assessment of fitness for surgery, and preparation of the uterus. This is followed by intraoperative care which includes antibiotic prophylaxis, antithrombotic measures, body fluid management, and body temperature management. Immediate postsurgical care involving the monitoring of vital parameters, pain management, care for vomiting, fluid balance, ambulation, antithrombotic measures, antibiotics, and wound and urinary catheter management are described. This chapter draws attention to the exclusion of specific organ injury, venous thromboembolism, surgical complications of haemorrhage, wound infection, urinary tract infection, and intestinal obstruction.

This excellent book comprehensively covers the knowledge needed for the performance of hysterectomy for benign conditions with a patient-centered focus. The author addresses with great detail the needs, merits, and demerits of each procedure followed by the careful, stepwise approach required to avoid complications. The chapters are not only well illustrated with color photographs for each step described but also furnished with a comprehensive list of references. I would highly recommend the book to practising gynecologist, and those in training. In addition, it is to a book to be made available in the theatre and in library of hospitals providing gynaecology services.

Sir Sabaratnam Arulkumaran PhD DSc FRCS FRCOG
Professor Emeritus of Obstetrics & Gynaecology
St George's, University of London, UK.
Past President of the Royal College of Obstetricians & Gynaecologists,
The British Medical Association & the International Federation of
Obstetrics & Gynaecology

May 1, 2021

1

Hysterectomy — What and Why

Introduction

Hysterectomy is one of the commonest major surgeries performed on women. In the United States of America, the Centers for Disease Control and Prevention (CDC) reported that, between 2006 and 2010, 11% of women in the age band of 40–44 years old and one third of women by the age of 60 years old had had a hysterectomy. Understandably, hysterectomy is one of the core surgical techniques that all residents in gynecology training would have to master early in their career.

This chapter explains the origins of the term "hysterectomy" and the different types of hysterectomy in current practice. The rationale for indications of hysterectomy is discussed at length in place of the common practice of providing a long and comprehensive list of uterine conditions for which hysterectomy may be performed. The educational goal of this chapter focuses on training the logical reasoning of young gynecologists to improve their confidence in making independent professional decisions on hysterectomy. This is to prepare them to adapt hysterectomy to the rapidly changing environment of technological advances, new understanding of pathophysiology of uterine conditions, medical innovations, and pharmaco-therapeutic developments.

It is an important part of patient care for a gynecologist to present the potential short-term and long-term outcomes of the surgery to women. This chapter explores the common consequences or physical changes in women after hysterectomy. The information assists gynecologists in discussion with women to reach an informed decision on hysterectomy.

What is Hysterectomy?

One may wonder why some surgical terms for operations involving the uterus carry the root word of "uterus", such as in "uterolysis" and "uteropexy", but the procedure to

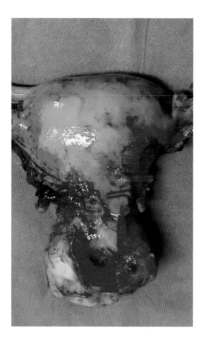

Figure 1.1 ■ A surgical photograph of a uterus removed by hysterectomy.

remove the uterus is called a hysterectomy (Figure 1.1). In ancient medical history, Greek physicians often made a diagnosis of hysteria for a myriad of female ailments and they ascribed the cause of hysteria to an unstable or wandering uterus. Thus emerged the medical term "hysteria" from the original word "hystera", which means uterus in Greek. In Anglo-Saxonized medical terminology, "hystera" for the uterus was retained while a suffix "-ectomy", referring to a surgical excision procedure in English, was added to form the term "hysterectomy" to describe the operation to remove the uterus. In the 20th century, medical terms for newly described surgical procedures adopt more common anatomical names, such as uteropexy.

When is Hysterectomy Indicated?

The sole indication for proposing to a woman that she should consider a hysterectomy is when the doctor has reached a conclusion that the surgery would improve her health status more than the potential detrimental consequences of the act, both immediately and in the long-term.

It is important to understand that a doctor's proposal of a treatment plan remains to be accepted by the patient who possesses sufficient cognitive capability to make her own decision. The concept of patient autonomy has a long history that can be traced back to Hippocrates (460–370 BC). Its role in current medical practice is further institutionalized legally. The indication to perform hysterectomy is therefore a legitimized collective decision between the gynecologist and the patient.

Factors influencing a gynecologist's decision on hysterectomy are grouped into pro-hysterectomy factors and anti-hysterectomy factors. Modern standard practice demands that gynecologists collect and appraise these factors objectively and without biases so that the decision on whether or not to propose a hysterectomy is deemed competent.

Pro-hysterectomy Factors

Uterine conditions giving rise to anatomical or physiological abnormalities that are objectively shown to be sufficiently threatening to the well-being of a patient's physical or mental health status are pro-hysterectomy factors. These include pathology that cannot be adequately managed without removal of the uterus and other factors where the severity of the condition poses a potential grave consequence to the well-being of the woman. The common factors, not an exhaustive list, are provided below:

Primary malignancy of the reproductive organs

Primary malignancy of the uterus, cervix, and ovary accounts for almost 20% of all cancers in women. Early cancers of these organs can be successfully controlled or cured by surgical extirpation of the primary organ. In locally advanced cancer, removal of the primary organ and its adjacent structures plays an important role in controlling and favorably altering the natural course of these cancers.

Secondary malignancy involving the uterus

Metastatic cancer from primary colorectal, stomach, and breast cancer are sometimes found on the ovary, uterus, and less commonly the cervix. Hysterectomy, in addition to resolving symptoms of the metastatic tumor, forms a part of the integral strategy for primary cancer management.

Uterine fibroids with complications

Uterine fibroid or leiomyoma is the commonest benign tumor in the female. It is found in at least 50% of women by the age of 40 years. More than 60% of uterine leiomyomas are innocent (i.e., without any symptoms) and do not require any medical interventions. The most significant common complication of leiomyoma is heavy menstrual bleeding leading to severe iron deficiency anemia. Other symptoms related to the space-occupying nature of the enlarged uterus by the leiomyoma include compression of the urinary bladder resulting in increased urinary frequency or voiding difficulty, and mass effect on the bowel causing constipation. Infrequently, leiomyoma that occupies the entire pelvic cavity, by compressing on the venous blood circulation coursing through the pelvis, causes venous thrombosis that carries a risk of life-threatening thromboembolism.

Symptomatic or large leiomyoma is the most common reason for hysterectomy for benign conditions.

Uterine adenomyosis

Uterine adenomyosis is an estrogen and progesterone-responsive condition of women of reproductive age. The incidence is higher in Asians than in Caucasians, and it induces uterine enlargement, heavy menstrual bleeding, and dysmenorrhea. When hormone-based therapy fails to control the symptoms adequately, hysterectomy confers a permanent cure for the condition.

Idiopathic heavy menstrual bleeding

Some women who experience periodic heavy menstrual bleeding do not have a detectable organic uterine pathology, a condition that was termed dysfunctional uterine bleeding in older textbooks. It has been a commonly documented reason for hysterectomy.

Uterine prolapse

Pelvic organ prolapse is a common disorder among post-menopausal women. In some cases, the uterus can prolapse beyond the introitus. Hysterectomy forms part of the corrective or reconstructive surgery of the pelvic floor structure to withhold the pelvic viscera.

Chronic pelvic pain

Chronic pelvic pain affects almost 20% of women. Hysterectomy is sometimes performed when the pain shows features of predominant uterine origin.

Postpartum hemorrhage

Severe postpartum hemorrhage is a significant cause of maternal mortality worldwide. A timely hysterectomy is a life-saving procedure.

Sexual reassignment

Hysterectomy is performed in female to male sexual reassignment procedure.

Uterine donation

Uterine transplantation has recently been shown to harbor successful pregnancy and has established a definitive role in organ transplantation programs. Hysterectomy is performed on the donor of the uterus.

Patient's constitution is fit for surgery

Hysterectomy is a major surgical procedure. Intraoperative or early postoperative complications may arise from blood loss, surgical infection, or cardiogenic or neurogenic disorders. Constitutional fitness is therefore a prerequisite factor for hysterectomy.

Anti-hysterectomy Factors

The mere presence of a uterine condition that is objectively found to be severely impacting a woman's health is insufficient on its own to justify a hysterectomy. A balanced appraisal of all factors must conclude that anti-hysterectomy factors are less than the pro-hysterectomy factors before a hysterectomy can be proposed to the woman for consideration. Again, without being exhaustive, the list below outlines the common anti-hysterectomy factors.

Available alternative management is efficacious

— Medical therapies such as estrogen, progesterone, nonsteroidal anti-inflammatory drugs, and anti-plasminogenic drugs have been found to be efficacious in the treatment of heavy menstrual bleeding with or without anemia, dysmenorrhea, or chronic pelvic pain.

Myometrial progesterone receptor inhibitors and gonadotropin-releasing hormone agonists and antagonists have proved to be efficacious in reducing both the size of leiomyoma and severity of heavy menstrual bleeding.

— Non-hysterectomy surgical procedures
Myomectomy is a well-established procedure for the treatment of heavy menstrual bleeding, dysmenorrhea, and visceral compressive complications related to uterine leiomyoma.

— Hysteroscopy-directed and non-hysteroscopy-directed endometrial ablation techniques have been available for almost three decades for the efficacious management of heavy menstrual bleeding related to submucous leiomyoma and idiopathic conditions.

— Interventional radiological uterine embolization
Uterine arteries and main vessels supplying a leiomyoma can be identified on angiography through interventional radiography techniques. Embolization of these arteries results in necrosis and reduction in dimension of the leiomyoma. It has been shown to be efficacious in managing complications from leiomyoma in some cases.

— Magnetic resonance imaging-directed high-frequency ultrasound ablation
Magnetic resonance imaging-directed application of focused high-frequency ultrasound energy has been shown to be efficacious in inducing necrosis and subsequent fibrosis in leiomyoma of appropriate dimensions.

Fertility preservation

The uterus is absolutely necessary for pregnancy. For women who want to preserve their fertility potential, hysterectomy is contraindicated.

Conscience

Hysterectomy, by removal of the organ unique to women, is against the conscience of some women. They see the cessation of menstruation as a loss of physiologic function and feminine sexuality. Some take the view that loss of an organ, diseased or not, infringes the integrity of their body and soul.

Physical and mental fitness

Concurrent medical morbidities known to increase the risk of serious surgical-anesthetic complications are anti-hysterectomy factors. For premenopausal women, coexisting medical conditions that contraindicate the postoperative use of estrogen replacement therapy should also be seen as an anti-hysterectomy factor.

Indecision/no consent

A woman's indecision on hysterectomy, regardless of her own reasons, is an important anti-hysterectomy factor since her informed consent is a necessity for the procedure.

Consequence of Hysterectomy

Hysterectomy is a common surgery among women. Doctors, whether gynecologists or otherwise, should know the consequences of hysterectomy so that they can provide patients with comprehensive care. Some of these consequences are real while others, either perceived or observed, do not have a causal relationship to hysterectomy.

Resolution of Pathology

Hysterectomy, by removing the uterus, resolves primarily and permanently uterine pathology, heavy menstrual bleeding, and dysmenorrhea. Research on patient outcomes has shown that more than 90% of patients were satisfied with hysterectomy. Existing evidence shows that hysterectomy is a cost-effective treatment for managing benign uterine conditions in many communities of varying socioeconomic status.

In selected cases where hysterectomy is performed for uterine malignancy, further oncological therapy may be needed to consolidate the overall cancer control.

Infertility

Hysterectomy, by nature, terminates the patient's fertility permanently, though this consequence can now be relieved with uterine transplantation in suitable women.

Amenorrhea and Menopause

The uterus is the source of menstruation, which is a periodic shedding of superficial endometrium in a nonpregnant state. Hysterectomy naturally induces amenorrhea. It carries no adverse health effects on women because menstruation has no physiological role other than reflecting the status of the pituitary-ovarian-endometrial axis. In this sense, endometrial shedding is the result of absence of pregnancy and can be seen as the "weeping of a disappointed womb".

Toward the end of reproductive life for women with an intact uterus, amenorrhea reflects cessation of estrogen and progesterone secretion from primary physiological ovarian failure. There may be estrogen deficiency symptoms and genital tract atrophy. Hysterectomy induces immediate menopause only if the surgery also removes the ovaries.

Some reports from observational studies estimate that hysterectomy brings forward ovarian menopause by up to three years earlier than the average age of menopause in the natural population, though the evidence is not conclusive. The mechanism for this phenomenon is thought to be related to an interruption of anastomotic blood circulation between the uterus and ovaries during hysterectomy. This argument is tenuous as the ovaries derive their primary blood supply directly from the aorta.

Sexual Dysfunction/Dyspareunia

It is a common cross-cultural perception among men and women that the uterus is related to femininity and sexual function. Good and convincing clinical data indicate that both male and female sexual satisfaction improves after hysterectomy by resolving the primary uterine pathology.

Deep dyspareunia and postcoital bleeding occur in a small number of women following hysterectomy, particularly during the early phase of postoperative recovery. The pain is the result of vaginal vault infection or hematoma. It usually resolves either after antibiotic treatment or spontaneously in less severe cases.

There is no significant shortening of the vagina following a simple total hysterectomy. In radical hysterectomy for cervical cancer, the upper 3 to 4 cm of the vagina is excised with the uterus. There may be a temporary dyspareunia. The vagina will lengthen to accommodate normal coitus after an interval of vaginal sexual intercourse.

Urinary Incontinence

Hysterectomy for large uterine mass tends to improve urinary frequency, urgency, mild urinary incontinence, and voiding difficulty.

Apart from rare surgical complications of ureterovaginal or vesicovaginal fistulation, urinary incontinence can occur as a consequence of cystitis from urinary catheterization in the perioperative period of hysterectomy. Voiding difficulty with overflow incontinence is sometimes seen during the postoperative period of radical hysterectomy because of urinary bladder denervation.

It is important to note that urinary incontinence in the pelvic organ prolapse syndrome may continue after hysterectomy, but not as a consequence of hysterectomy.

Constipation

Constipation is a common symptom among women, with or without existence of the uterus. In the immediate postoperative recovery phase, constipation is related to the intraoperative manipulation of bowels or a result of anticholinergic properties of some medications. These situations are self-limiting and short-lived.

Long-term constipation occasionally complicates radical hysterectomy because of rectal denervation.

Vaginal Prolapse

The main support of the uterus is the pelvic diaphragm, aided by cardinal and uterosacral ligaments. These structures also support the vaginal vault through the extended fibers that are inserted directly into the vagina. Most women with pelvic organ prolapse have an intact uterus. The main cause of prolapse is neuromuscular damage to the pelvic diaphragm and pelvic ligaments from pregnancy and childbirth, aggravated by genital tract atrophy from estrogen deficiency.

Unlike radical hysterectomy, hysterectomy for benign uterine conditions involves dissection of cardinal and uterosacral ligaments close to the cervix and incision of the pelvic diaphragm limited to the vaginal fornix. These procedures cause no or negligible disruption to the integrity of the pelvic diaphragm and supportive ligaments of the vagina. Furthermore, the stumps of severed ligaments are adhered to the vaginal vault by surgical sutures during vaginal vault closure. It is uncommon for women without preexisting defects in the pelvic diaphragm to develop vaginal prolapse following a simple hysterectomy.

Lower Limb Lymphedema

The incidence of lymphedema following a radical hysterectomy with comprehensive bilateral pelvic lymphadenectomy ranges between 5% and 10%. In the majority of cases, the severity is mild and the patient experiences heaviness in the lower lymph after a long walk, particularly towards end of day. Severe lymphedema presenting with lower limb swelling, increase girth of the calf muscles occurs in 1% of these cases.

Post-hysterectomy Syndrome

This is an old term that is used to describe a small number of women who, after hysterectomy, complain of a highly variable group of symptoms that are largely psychoemotional in nature. Its existence as an entity has been dismissed. Some of the symptoms are related to persistence of premenstrual syndrome or preexisting emotional and affective disorders. Included in this group of women are those who experience estrogen deficiency due to menopause, with or without bilateral oophorectomy.

Types of Hysterectomy

Method of hysterectomy and the extent of tissue removed during hysterectomy have been evolving with technological improvements, advancements in our understanding of pathology, development of surgical expertise, improvements in medicine and anesthesia that enhance the safety of surgery, and changes in women's expectations and demands. The choice of the method of hysterectomy has moved away from being guided by the surgeon's experience and preference to evidence-based practice.

The type of hysterectomy is classified by mode of surgical access to the uterus and according to the extent of surgery.

Classification by Mode of Surgical Access to the Uterus

— Abdominal hysterectomy: Hysterectomy performed through a laparotomy;
— Vaginal hysterectomy: The entire surgical process is completed through the vagina;
— Laparoscopic total hysterectomy: The entire hysterectomy is completed laparoscopically, and the uterus is retrieved via the vagina or through laparoscopic incision after organ morcellation;
— Laparoscopy-assisted vaginal hysterectomy: Surgery on the supra-vaginal portion of the uterus is performed laparoscopically and the cervical portion is performed through the vagina.
— Robotic Hysterectomy: In this surgery, robotic technology replaces the traditional laparoscopy for access to the uterus.

Classification According to Surgical Extent

The extent of surgical excision for the uterus includes extirpation of the entire uterus, which includes the uterine corpus and cervix, or limited excision of the uterine corpus alone. Furthermore, excision of the uterus can be combined with excision of the uterine appendages, the Fallopian tubes, and the ovaries.

Salpingectomy

The Fallopian tubes are the ductal structures for transportation of ova and sperms, and the ampulla regions are the sites where fertilization of the ovum occurs. The luminal epithelium of the Fallopian tubes is secretory of serous fluid. Fallopian tubes carry no hormonal functions.

During hysterectomy, the Fallopian tubes are occluded at the uterine ends. The serous secretion is discharged into the peritoneal cavity via the fimbrial terminals. Postsurgical scarring and adhesions often result in partial or complete occlusion of the fimbrial terminals, leading to formation of hydrosalpinx for which some women may need to undergo a second surgery. Recent evidence showed that epithelium of the Fallopian tubes is the site of origin for high-grade serous adenocarcinoma, in particular the type of adenocarcinoma related to the inherited pathologic variants of mutations in breast cancer genes BRCA-1 and BRCA-2.

Bilateral salpingectomy during hysterectomy has no discernable additional alteration in a woman's physiology, but it prevents second surgery for symptomatic hydrosalpinx and would reduce the incidence of serous adenocarcinoma of the Fallopian tubes. Bilateral salpingectomy is now recommended and widely practiced during all hysterectomy.

Oophorectomy

The ovaries are the organs contributing more than 99% of all the circulatory estrogens and progesterone in premenopausal women. They also secrete and contribute to 25% of circulatory androgens in women. The androgen secretory function of the ovaries continues for a number of years beyond natural menopause. Bilateral oophorectomy renders menopausal women with deficiencies in estrogens, progesterone, and androgens. The impact of hormonal deficiencies on women's health is profound and long lasting.

The proximity of the ovaries to the uterus and the seemingly imminent menopause are not reasons for any surgeon to remove them during hysterectomy. It is an absolute necessity, not a mere prudence or an exercise of due diligence, for surgeons to discuss with the woman on the role of oophorectomy during hysterectomy for benign conditions.

Thus, the extent of surgery can be used to classify hysterectomy into the following types:

— **Total hysterectomy (TH)**: This is a surgery to remove the entire uterus, which includes both the corpus and the cervix (Figure 1.1).
— **Total hysterectomy with bilateral salpingectomy (THBS)**: In this procedure, the right and left Fallopian tubes are removed with hysterectomy (Figure 1.2a).
— **Total hysterectomy with salpingo-oophorectomy**: This is a simple total hysterectomy with removal of the Fallopian tube and ovary (Figures 1.2b,c). Salpingo-oophorectomy (SO) can be right (RSO), left (LSO), or both sides (BSO).

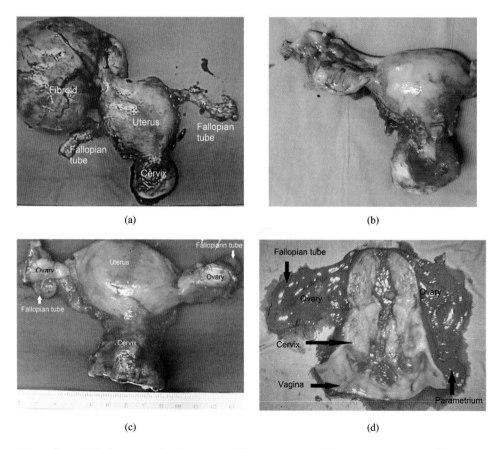

Figure 1.2 ■ Surgical photographs showing different types of hysterectomy in addition to a total hysterectomy. (a): Total hysterectomy with bilateral salpingectomy; (b) total hysterectomy with unilateral salpingo-oophorectomy; (c) total hysterectomy with bilateral salpingo-oophorectomy; and (d) radical hysterectomy.

— **Subtotal hysterectomy**: The prefix "sub-" denotes "less than". Therefore, "subtotal" is used in contrast to "total" in hysterectomy. This limited surgery removes the uterine corpus while leaving behind the cervix.

— **Radical hysterectomy (RH):** This is a surgery for uterine malignancy and, in particular, cervical cancer. In addition to the uterus, the surgery further removes a length of the proximal parametrium and vagina (Figure 1.2d). This is often accompanied with dissection of regional pelvic lymph nodes (lymphadenectomy) and may be combined with excision of the Fallopian tubes and/or ovaries on a case-by-case basis.

In practice, the type of hysterectomy for benign conditions is described by combining the two classifications with ramifications:

	Method of Access to the Uterus		
Extent of surgery	**Laparotomy**	**Laparoscopy**	**Vaginal**
Uterus only, entire organ (total)	TAH	LTH	VH
+ Fallopian tubes	TAH + BS	LTH + BS	VH + BS
+ ovary, right	TAH + RSO	LTH + RSO	VH + RSO
+ ovary, left	TAH + LSO	LTH + LSO	VH + LSO
+ ovaries, both sides	TAH + BSO	LTH + BSO	VH + BSO
Uterus, corpus only (subtotal)	STH	LSH	—
+ Fallopian tubes	SH + BS	LSH + BS	—
+ ovary, right	SH + RSO	LSH + RSO	—
+ ovary, left	SH + LSO	LSH + LSO	—
+ ovaries, both sides	SH + BSO	LSH + BSO	—

	Laparoscopy and vaginal combined
Uterus only, entire organ (total)	LAVH
+ Fallopian tubes	LAVH + BS
+ ovary, right	LAVH + RSO
+ ovary, left	LAVH + LSO
+ ovaries, both sides	LAVH + BSO

TAH = total abdominal hysterectomy; TLH = laparoscopic total hysterectomy; VH = vaginal hysterectomy; BS = bilateral salpingectomy; RSO = right salpingo-oophorectomy; LSO = left salpingo-oophorectomy; BSO = bilateral salpingo-oophorectomy; LAVH = laparoscopy-assisted vaginal hysterectomy.

References

Broder MS, Kanouse DE, Mittman BS, *et al.* (2000) The appropriateness of recommendations for hysterectomy. *Obstet Gynecol* **95**(2): 199–205. doi: 10.1016/s0029-7844(99)00519-0.

Burger HG. (2002) Androgen production in women. *Fertil Steril* **77**(Suppl 4): S3–5. doi: 10.1016/s0015-0282(02)02985-0.

Clarke-Pearson DL, Geller EJ. (2013) Complications of hysterectomy. *Obstet Gynecol* **121**: 654–673.

Corona LE, Swenson CW, Sheetz KH, *et al.* (2015) Use of other treatments before hysterectomy for benign conditions in a statewide hospital collaborative. *Am J Obstet Gynecol* **212**(3): 304.e1–7. doi: 10.1016/j.ajog.2014.11.031. Epub 2014 Dec 23.

Emerson J, Paquet A, Sangha R, *et al.* (2019) Gynecologic surgical outcomes through the patient's eyes: are physicians looking in the same direction? *Obstet Gynecol Surv* **74**(6): 351–361. doi: 10.1097/OGX.0000000000000681.

Garry R. (2005) Health economics of hysterectomy. *Best Pract Res Clin Obstet Gynaecol* **19**(3): 451–465. doi: 10.1016/j.bpobgyn.2005.01.010. Epub 2005 Mar 2.

Laughlin-Tommaso SK, Khan Z, Weaver AL, *et al.* (2018) Cardiovascular and metabolic morbidity after hysterectomy with ovarian conservation: a cohort study. *Menopause* **25**(5): 483–492.

Lykke R, Blaakær J, Ottesen B, *et al.* (2015) The indication for hysterectomy as a risk factor for subsequent pelvic organ prolapse repair. *Int Urogynecol J* **26**(11):1661–1665. doi: 10.1007/s00192-015-2757-y. Epub 2015 Jun 7.

Solnik MJ, Munro MG. (2014) Indications and alternatives to hysterectomy. *Clin Obstet Gynecol* **57**(1): 14–42. doi: 10.1097/GRF.0000000000000010.

Taipale K, Leminen A, Räsänen P, *et al.* (2009) Costs and health-related quality of life effects of hysterectomy in patients with benign uterine disorders. *Acta Obstet Gynecol Scand* **88**(12): 1402–1410. doi: 10.3109/00016340903317990.

Thurston J, Murji A, Scattolon S, *et al.* (2019) No. 377-hysterectomy for benign gynaecologic indications. *J Obstet Gynaecol Can* **41**(4): 543–557. doi: 10.1016/j.jogc.2018.12.006.

2

Laparotomy for Hysterectomy

Introduction

Laparotomy with a midline incision on the anterior abdominal wall, a generic surgical technique in general abdominal surgery, has been adopted as the method of accessing the uterus in the pelvis since hysterectomy was first performed in 1843 by Dr Charles Clay in Manchester, England. It provides good surgical exposure for inspection, examination, and manipulation of pelvic structures and is suitable for extirpation of the uterus afflicted by any pathology, benign or malignant. Surgical techniques have since changed significantly, resulting in many surgical approaches for accessing the pelvis for hysterectomy today.

The content of this chapter focuses on (1) the rationale and basis of choosing the type of laparotomy incision that is optimal for hysterectomy and (2) the surgical technique in laparotomy incisions. The detail of anatomy and basis of physiology in the development of different laparotomy incisions is cornerstone in enforcing the intellectual reasoning of gynecologists in selecting one incision over the other, equipping them with sound approaches to deal with any unintended or unanticipated operative encounters, and raising their curiosity and interest in the further development of abdominal surgical techniques.

Midline Laparotomy

Median abdominal incision is a classical way of opening an abdominal cavity that fits all types of surgical pathology. The potential for extending the incision any way between the pubis below and xiphisternum above allows surgeons to open an abdominal wall aperture of varying size as necessitated by the pathology.

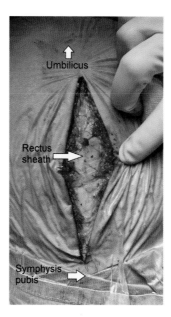

Figure 2.1 ■ A surgical photograph showing a subumbilical midline incision.

For gynecological surgeries confined to pathology within the pelvis and lower part of the abdomen, the incision is placed below the umbilicus, often referred to as a subumbilical midline incision (Figure 2.1).

With knowledge of the anatomy of the abdomen wall acquired early during surgical training, most residents believe that this type of incision does not demand a high level of psychomotor dexterity. It is an incision that one learns from the demonstration of an operating surgeon and doing it oneself intuitively through the modus operandi of "see one, do one, teach one". Nonetheless, the nuances of the incision are best illustrated in challenging encounters, of which less experienced gynecologists sometimes require assistance from the senior surgeons.

"A Deep Pelvis"

In obstetrics, I learned the Caldwell-Moloy classification of the capacity and shape of pelvis according to four types: Gynecoid, anthropoid, android, and platypelloid. The round and symmetrical gynecoid pelvis is the most favorable for vaginal birth. The android or male type pelvis with a triangular inlet, narrow pelvic outlet, and small acute angle of pubic arch is the least favorable. When one performs a hysterectomy and approaches the pelvis from the abdominal cavity, a gynecoid and platypelloid pelvis has a wide inlet that makes the uterus easily accessible for extirpation. An android or anthropoid pelvis, on the other hand, is either narrow and tapering toward the pelvic floor or cylindrical in shape and appearing deep and narrow, which constrains surgical maneuvers on the lower pedicles during hysterectomy. The expression "deep pelvis" is often used when reporting this surgical challenge. This surgical difficulty is accentuated, and sometimes artificially created, by a midline abdominal incision that ends too far above the pubic symphysis. Extension of the abdominal incision toward the pubis increases the incision aperture, causing the apparent "deep" pelvis to disappear.

"How Long is the Skin Incision?"

Patients told of a midline incision often ask about the length of the skin incision. They are generally satisfied with the answer, "long enough for me to do the hysterectomy safely for you". The length of abdominal wound incision should be tailored to the dimensions of the uterus. Overzealous incision is associated with increased blood loss and incidence of surgical wound infection.

Considering the accessibility of the pelvis and that the dimensions of the uterus do not extend to a level above the umbilicus, a midline incision that spans from 2 cm below the umbilicus to 1 cm above the superior border of the symphysis pubis is adequate for most cases of hysterectomy.

"The Bloody Wound"

The cutis layer of skin, white and fibrous when incised using a sharp scalpel, is relatively bloodless. The subcutaneous layer of adipose tissue is then incised with an electro-diathermy pen over the entire length of the surgical wound to expose the anterior rectus sheath. Any bleeding points encountered can be sealed with diathermy immediately.

Bothersome bleedings are often encountered at the apex of surgical incisions due to the vascular networks of capillaries present. Nameless in anatomical terms, these capillary vessels are what I call the "angular vein of assault" that contributes to bothersome bleeding during surgery. If not adequately controlled, they can lead to postoperative surgical wound hematoma, infection, and pain.

A midline abdominal incision allows the abdominal cavity to be directly entered after dividing the linea alba, which binds the right and left rectus abdominis muscles at the midline. The blood supply to linea alba are delivered via capillaries from each rectus abdominis, but the capillaries stop at the midline without communication between the vascular beds of the two sides. The anatomical divide results in a relatively avascular central line in the linea alba (Figures 2.2).

Once linea alba is incised, the right and left recti abdominis muscles are gently separated. Excessive retraction on the muscles can rupture perforating blood vessels causing excessive bleeding.

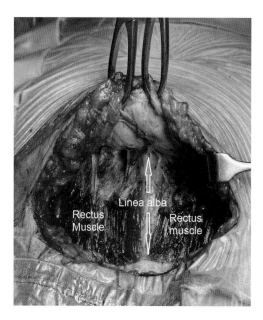

Figure 2.2 ■ The avascular linea alba is shown in this surgical photograph taken during a Pfannenstiel incision.

"The Obscure Linea Alba"

The linea alba is where the right and left rectus abdominis muscles meet at the midline of the anterior abdominal wall. Incision of the linea alba is necessary for separation of the muscles to expose the anterior peritoneum. The identification of this line where the fibrous tissue fuses is sometimes indistinct. Inadvertent separation of longitudinally running muscle fiber bundles in the belly of the rectus abdominis invariably causes more bleeding into the wound. Tips for avoiding this difficulty include:

— Placing two Kocher forceps a short distance apart along the edge of the ipsilateral incision of the linea alba. A sharp scalpel is used to scrape, not cut, the muscle fibers away from under the surface of the tautly held rectus sheath.
— If incision of the wound, including the anterior sheath, has been adequately made toward the pubis, one should see the two pyramidalis muscles immediately anterior to the rectus abdominis (Figure 2.3), which are two small triangular muscles with the base located at the pubis. The apex of the right and left pyramidalis muscles extends upward and converges toward the midline. The direction of the two small muscles effectively works as an arrow pointing to the midline of the fusion of the rectus abdominis muscles.

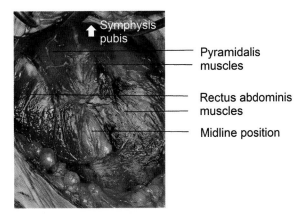

Figure 2.3 ■ A surgical photograph showing the direction of the apex of two pyramidalis muscles converging on the linea alba.

"Scalpel versus Scissors"

After separating the rectus abdominis below the arcuate line (also known as the semicircular line of Douglas) at the midpoint between the pubic crest and umbilicus, the thin fascia transversalis is held up with artery forceps and incised to expose the anterior parietal peritoneum, which in turn is incised to enter the abdominal cavity. A sharp scalpel allows these two thin layers of tissue to be incised separately. Scalpel incision is linear and extends superficially toward the deeper layer, permitting direct visualization of tissues being incised. Some surgeons enter the cavity by incising the two layers together with scissors. Incision with scissors involves cutting across a fold of tissue through and through in a single movement, which will cut through any tissues within the little fold of incision. Unintended enterotomy will result if a small part of bowel loop is inadvertently included within the fold of the peritoneum.

Failure to Reach Abdominal Cavity

On puncturing the peritoneum, there is an immediate and sudden falling back of the intestines below the held up peritoneum as air rushes into the abdominal cavity.

There are occasions where entering the abdominal cavity is not so straightforward, particularly in the presence of adhesions from prior surgeries or when the omentum is adherent to the anterior parietal peritoneum. There may be difficulty in recognizing the adipose tissue of omentum from extraperitoneal fatty tissue. If the incision wound is not heavily stained by blood, these adipose tissues are distinguishable by color. The preperitoneal adipose tissue is yellow or amber whereas the omental adipose tissue appears pale yellow.

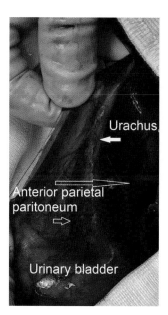

Figure 2.4 ■ A surgical photograph showing the urachus.

Awareness of the patient's prior surgery is helpful for the surgeon in predicting the probable site of adhesions and in choosing the most appropriate site of peritoneal incision either in the upper or lower part of the abdomen.

The Urachus

On extending the incision of the anterior parietal peritoneum toward the pelvis, one would meet a whitish fibrous band of tissue on the peritoneum at the midline location (Figure 2.4), which can be traced to the dorm of the urinary bladder. This is a median umbilical ligament, a remnant structure of the urachus. The urachus of the allantois is an embryonic canal that drains urine from the bladder to the umbilical cord. Anatomically, this is situated between the transversalis fascia anteriorly and the peritoneum posteriorly.

It is recommended that one should avoid transecting the ligament as a rare complication of urinary fistula or sinus may result in rare cases of patent urachus. Paying attention to this ligament toward the urinary bladder will also help in identifying the dorm of the bladder and, thus, helps to prevent any inadvertent urinary bladder cystotomy.

Closure of the Vertical Midline Incision

Closure of surgical wound is needed to achieve healing by primary intention. Mass closure in a single layer is the recommended method of closing midline abdominal incisions. Surgical technique and choice of suture material affect the healing process, quality, and integrity of the wound and long-term outcome of the structure of the abdominal wound.

The choice of suture depends on whether the wound is clean or contaminated, the length of incision, the patient's constitutional state, and the suture's characteristics, such as the material composition's absorbability, tensile strength, and handling property. The most commonly used sutures for closure of a midline wound for hysterectomy are poly-dioxanone (PDS) and nylon to ensure a prolonged period of dermal support in the process of wound healing. PDS is an absorbable suture that is degraded by hydrolysis. It retains tensile strength very well, specifically 74% at day-14, 58% at day-28, and 41% at week-6 after surgery. Nylon is a nonabsorbable synthetic suture. When buried in the tissue, it loses its tensile strength slowly and remains almost at 100% up to 6 months after surgery. Compared to PDS, nylon has poor handling property and low security of knots, which require more throws during knot tying.

The closure of the wound commences at its apex near the umbilicus. This a critical anchoring suture point that must include the entire thickness of the rectus sheath. Careful attention is needed here to prevent the suture from piercing the fibrotic tissue of the umbilicus as the position of the umbilicus may be distorted or, if the suture pierces through the umbilical skin, wound infection or sinus formation may occur.

The remaining opening in the rectus sheath is then closed with continuously locking sutures placed 1 cm from the edge and 1 cm in between stitches until the apex of the incision above the symphysis pubis. The last stitch should secure the apex closure completely to prevent bleeding from the "angular vein of assault" and to avoid leaving a gap in the sheath which would predispose the wound to herniation. There are two helpful maneuvers that one can employ. The common method is to use a pair of artery forceps to hold up the apex at the beginning of the wound closure to allow the closing suture to be placed beyond it. The other method is to hold the last 2 or 3 continuous stitches loosely so that the apex can be accessed easily. Once the last stitch has been placed, the continuous stitches are tightened to close the sheath completely.

The surgeon's square knot at the end of the suture tends to be quite thick. It is sometimes felt as a tender subcutaneous nodule or a lump that is noticeable to slim patients whose subcutaneous adipose layer is thin. The risk of this occurrence can be mitigated by burying the knot in deeper layers of tissue. This is done by holding the needle end of the suture taut and, from a point immediately distal to the knot, pass the needle below the rectus sheath in a reverse direction toward the umbilicus over a distance of 2 cm. The needle is picked up and, by pulling the suture, the thick knot will be inverted and buried below the sheath.

Closure of subcutaneous adipose tissue is unnecessary. Skin can be closed with continuous subcuticular Vicryl sutures, interrupted vertical mattress sutures, or surgical staplers according to the surgeon's choice. Monocryl, an absorbable monofilament suture is widely used for this purpose.

Transverse Abdominal Incisions

Large abdominal incisions are associated with significant postoperative pain and complications such as pneumonia and thromboembolic phenomena associated with prolonged bed rest, as well as long-term risk of incisional herniation of abdominal viscera (Figure 2.5). In addition, some patients find the obvious scar in the middle of the abdomen unsightly and aesthetically unacceptable. Many surgeons have developed alternative incisions for abdominal surgeries to circumvent incisional hernia and improve the cosmetic appearance of surgical scars (Figure 2.6).

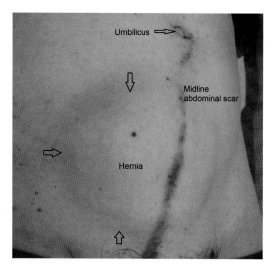

Figure 2.5 ■ A clinical photograph showing a large hernia in a midline laparotomy incision wound.

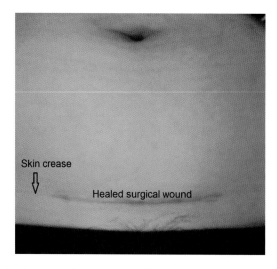

Figure 2.6 ■ A clinical photograph showing a healed transverse lower abdominal incision.

There are three well-described transverse abdominal incisions for pelvic surgeries: Pfannenstiel, Maylard, and Joel-Cohen incisions.

Pfannenstiel Incision

The first and most significant contribution to the development of the transverse abdominal incision came from Dr Herrmann Johannes Pfannenstiel, a German-born gynecologist who worked in Vienna. In 1900, he proposed a method of transverse incision along the skin crease just above the pubic hair line in a publication involving 51 cases of abdominal surgeries. He illustrated the procedure in a diagram in which the anterior abdominal wall was marked with a solid transverse line above the pubis and a dotted vertical line at the midline between the umbilicus and the pubis. The caption on the diagram reads, "die bogenformige tranversale linie bedeutet den Schnitt durch haut, unterhautferrgewebe und die fascien, die punktirte den Schnitt durch den die zwischen den musculi recto gelegene bindegewebsschnitt, die fascia transvera und das peritoneum" which, in English, means "the arch-shaped transverse line means the line through the skin, subcutaneous tissue, and the fascia, the dotted line means the incision through the connective tissue incision between the rectus abdominis muscles, the fascia transversalis, and peritoneum". Dr Pfannenstiel died of sepsis after a needle-stick injury to his finger while performing on a tubo-ovarian abscess in 1907. This incision, which has since become his namesake, was popularized in the English medical field in 1911 by Dr Monroe Kerr, an English gynecologist who spent his entire career in Glasgow, the United Kingdom. The incision has also been known as the Pfannenstiel-Kerr incision, or simply Kerr incision in England. It has since remained a popular approach to laparotomy for hysterectomy when the size of the uterus is normal or moderately enlarged, as well as for cesarean sections.

The Pfannenstiel incision, compared to a midline laparotomy, is famously known for its excellent aesthetic effect. The transverse skin incision located at about 2 cm above the superior border of the symphysis pubis is often concealed by pubic hair. The fibrous scar is inconspicuous along the natural skin crease and it is referred to in lay terms as a "bikini" scar. From a surgical outcome perspective, the transverse incision of the fascia, most notably the anterior rectal sheath, is the most significant deviation of the approach from a midline incision. A transverse incision is less traumatic to aponeurosis as it separates the fibers rather than cutting across them in a midline vertical incision. The pulling force on a transverse abdominal surgical wound is also significantly less than the midline wound. These two characteristics confer better tensile strength and integrity to transverse incisions than to midline vertical incisions.

Several considerations should be addressed when performing the Pfannenstiel incision:

Anatomical and physiological considerations in choosing the position of the Pfannenstiel incision

The definitive and fixed landmarks in the surgical surface anatomy of the anterior lower abdomen are the umbilicus superiorly, the symphysis pubis inferiorly, and the right and left anterior superior iliac spines laterally. The superior border of the pubic hairline in females is generally horizontal, but its position between the symphysis and the umbilicus is variable. Skin creases, if present, are along the Langer's lines which are oriented in a latero-medio-inferor direction. A transverse incision cuts along instead of across the transversely running fibrous fibres. The pulling force in the fibrous connective tissue in alignment with Langer's lines gives rise to the effect that the wound edges fall together naturally. In contrast, the transversely directed pulling force of transected fibrous connective tissue fibres in a vertical incision results in the skin edges being pulled apart to produce a gaping wound.

A standard Pfannenstiel incision is positioned 2 cm above the symphysis pubis and extended laterally toward but not up to the level of the anterior superior iliac spines, producing a symmetrical and slightly curved incision line resembling a smiling face. Some surgeons would ink the line of incision with a marker pen to ensure the best cosmetic benefit of the incision.

The incision is then extended transversely through the subcutaneous adipose tissues, cutting through the fatty Campa and slightly more fibrous Scappa fascia, until the anterior rectus sheath is reached.

Any bleeding points encountered on the incision are sealed with electrocautery. The superficial epigastric artery, which can be seen between the superficial fascia at the lateral end of the incision, is a branch of the femoral artery, courses upward to the level of the umbilicus, and supplies blood to the superficial abdominal wall. While it can be sealed off, it is preferably conserved by digital dissection of the adipose tissue at this point. The artery is used in the superficial epigastric flap in reconstructive surgery that requires a large amount of fatty tissue and skin.

Dissection of the anterior sheath

The anterior rectus sheath appears as a dense, whitish aponeurotic tissue. Two small transverse incisions are made 2 cm lateral to each side of the midline to expose the rectus abdominis muscles (Figure 2.7a). The two sheath incisions are then extended laterally toward the respective anterior superior iliac spine. This is best achieved by separating the sheath away from the underlying muscle before extending the incision of the sheath. Two Kocher forceps are used to lift the edges of the initial small sheath incision (Figure 2.7b). A closed Mayo scissor is inserted under the sheath and gently advanced toward the lateral end of the surgical wound. The scissor is then opened slightly to separate the sheath from the underlying rectus abdominis muscle. The sheath can then be incised with the scissor or electrodiathermy.

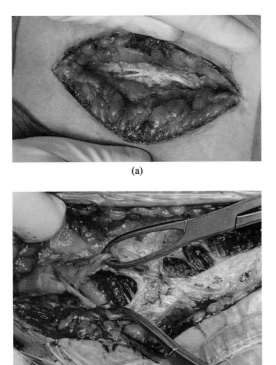

(a)

(b)

Figure 2.7 ■ Surgical photographs showing the opening of the rectus sheath from a Pfannenstiel incision.

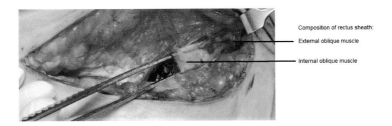

Figure 2.8 ■ A surgical photograph showing the opening of the lateral part of the rectus sheath by dividing the aponeurosis of the external and internal oblique muscles individually.

On incising the sheath toward the lateral end, one will witness the fibrous conjoint aponeurosis separating into its component aponeurosis of external and internal oblique muscles. The fibers of the internal oblique muscle, deep under the external oblique muscle, extend more medially than the external oblique muscles. The two aponeurosis should be opened individually to avoid cutting the medial muscle fibers of the internal oblique muscle (Figure 2.8). This maneuver reduces muscle bleeding and avoids the incorporation of muscle fibers in the wound closure, which is one of the causes of chronic wound pain from excessive fibrosis or neuroma formation.

Dissection of the anterior rectus sheath toward the umbilicus

Cephalad separation of a transversely incised anterior sheath from the rectus abdominis on both sides of the midline is necessary for the subsequent vertical separation of the recti abdominis muscles at the midline to achieve adequate incision aperture on the anterior abdominal wall. The exposure of a large area of muscles poses a unique surgical challenge when carrying out the Pfannenstiel incision. Bothersome bleeding often occurs from injury to muscle fibers and rupture of perforating blood vessels (Figure 2.9).

Surgeons should exercise their appreciation of the structural organization of muscle fibers. The basic unit of skeletal muscle is a muscle fiber wrapped in thin fibrous connective tissue known as endomysium. Several basic units are grouped in a bundle wrapped by a connective tissue layer, or perimysium, to form an intermediate units known as a fasciculus. Blood vessels and nerve fibers run between the fasciculi. The final structure of a named skeletal muscle is formed from the wrapping of a large number of muscle fasciculi by epimysium. In surgical encounters, epimysium is the first layer of the structure of skeletal muscle. The thin connective tissue of epimysium appear indistinct when it is stained by blood from the wound incision. Yet, surgical dissection that removes epimysium may injure the blood vessels between muscle fasciculi and result in excessive bleeding. Careful attention is needed when dissecting the anterior sheath to avoid injuring the epimysium of the rectus abdominis muscles (Figure 2.9).

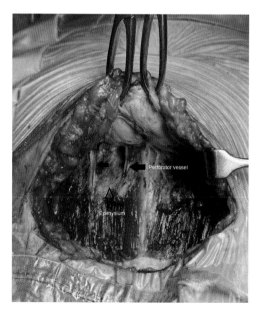

Figure 2.9 ■ A surgical photograph showing the process of revealing the upper flap of the rectus sheath.

In practice, the edge of the upper incision on the sheath is lifted with a pair of Kocher forceps and the rectus muscle is gently pushed away from the sheath between the median line of the muscle and midline of the abdomen, where the epimysium is least adherent to the anterior sheath. Perforator blood vessels encountered are sealed with electro-diathermy. The separation continues to the level just below the umbilicus. When the dissection is completed on both sides, two tunnels are created between the anterior sheath and the recti abdominis muscles along the fibrous linea alba. This is then cut with Mayo scissors or electrodiathermy to connect the two tunnels at the midline.

It is important to avoid unnecessary separation of the anterior sheath toward the lateral borders of the recti abdominis where increased vascular networks are located.

Opening of the anterior sheath toward the pubis

The extent of dissection of the anterior sheath toward the pubis symphysis depends on the distance of the wound incision away from the pubis. For a standard transverse incision 2 to 3 cm above the pubis, the dissection is minimal and is performed in the same manner as described for the cephalad dissection. Special attention is needed to avoid bleeding by injuring the pyramidalis muscles.

Risk of wound hematoma

One characteristic feature of the Pfannenstiel incision is the dead space created by the dissection of the rectus sheath from the underlying rectus abdominis. The abundance of perforator blood vessels running perpendicularly from the rectus abdominis muscles to the rectus sheath is a potential challenge to secure hemostasis and prevent incisional wound hematoma.

When the security of hemostasis is in doubt, as in cases where extensive dissection is performed after bad fibrosis from prior surgeries or when perioperative anticoagulation is planned, insertion of a closed suction drainage below the sheath is advisable for monitoring and management of wound bleeding in the immediate postoperative period.

Wound hematoma is an adverse surgical outcome that prolongs postoperative recovery time, causes severe wound pain, and gives rise to risk of wound infection and dehiscence. Surgeons should take all the precautions to prevent it.

Chronic pain in the Pfannenstiel incision wound

Although the cosmetic appearance of Pfannenstiel incisional scar is generally pleasing, it is not without incidence of keloid formation. To determine whether patients are satisfied with hysterectomy in the long term, my colleague and I conducted a study that was published in the *Australian and New Zealand Journal of Obstetrics and Gynaecology* in 1998. In a follow-up of 12 months or more of a group of 228 women who had laparotomy hysterectomy performed by a group of gynecologists at the Department of Obstetrics and Gynecology, Singapore General Hospital, 95.8% reported relief of their original symptoms but only 87% were satisfied with the operation. Pain in the abdominal wound a year or more after surgery was one of the most common reasons cited for dissatisfaction with hysterectomy.

Other investigators have reported chronic pain in Pfannenstiel wounds, mainly at the two ends of the wound or along the midline up to the level below the umbilicus. The painful spot below the umbilicus marks the upper end of the separation of the rectus abdominis muscles. Closure of the longitudinally incised parietal peritoneum is generally not recommended unless hemostasis necessitates it. The suture knot at the extreme of the wound may result in fibrosis, which causes nerve entrapment and chronic pain. This phenomenon is more prominent at the two extreme ends of a transversely incised anterior sheath where the sutures and suture knots are thick and aggravated by any incorporation of muscle fibers. The course of the iliohypogastric nerve (the thoracic nerve root T12 and lumbar nerve root 1) reaches a point 2 cm medial and 1 cm inferior to the anterior superior iliac spine, a position that may result in injuries by the incision. Neuromas in the post-operative period maybe a source of chronic wound pain.

Cutaneous numbness and paraesthesia in the lower abdomen

The sensory nerve supply of the lower abdomen derives from the iliohypogastric and ilioinguinal nerves (lumbar nerve roots L1 and L2). The terminal branches of the iliohypogastric nerve innervate the skin of the anterior abdomen halfway between the umbilicus and the pubis. The sensory branch of the ilioinguinal nerve innervates the abdominal wall 3 cm lateral to the midline and 2 cm above the symphysis pubis. The severance of these nerve fibers results in a sensation of numbness following surgery. Paraesthesia is the condition when numbness is accompanied by a tingling or pricking discomfort. Paraesthesia resulting from a Pfannenstiel incision is usually mild, unlike paraethesia from nerve root compression on the lateral femoral nerve where the paraesthesia over the lateral thigh on the affected side is described as meralgia paraesthesia.

Closure of the Pfannestiel incision

The incision edge of the parietal peritoneum is checked for secure hemostasis and placed together at the midline below the recti abdominis muscles. Hemostasis in the anterior sheath and the recti abdominis is confirmed. The wound is held open gently with

Langenbeck retractors to expose the end of the incision on the aponeurosis of oblique muscles. The two edges of the aponeurosis are picked up with a pair of tooth forceps, such as Bonney forceps, and secured with a figure-of-8 suture at the apex. The end of this suture is held on to a pair of mosquito forceps as an anchor suture. The same maneuver is performed at the other end of the wound and the same suture, in continuous stitches, is used to close the remaining incision of the sheath to meet the anchor suture. The suture is tied with the ends of the anchor suture using a secure surgeon's square knot.

Absorbable synthetic braided sutures are most commonly used for this purpose, with the most popular being polyglactin (Vicryl, size U.S.P 1) and polyglycolic acid (Dexon) sutures. Polyglactin sutures are degraded by hydrolysis and maintain 65% of the tensile strength at day-14. The rate of degradation is 90% after 28 days, and they are completely absorbed by day-100. Polyglycolic acid sutures are degraded predominantly by hydrolysis and, to a small extent, by enzymatic esterase activity. This suture loses 50% of its tensile strength by 2 weeks and 100% by four weeks, and is completely degraded by 90–120 days.

Closure of subcutaneous adipose tissue is unnecessary as the force of the wound brings the edges of skin together naturally. However, if a very thin suture or tissue glue is being used to close the skin and the adipose tissue layer is thick, I recommend closing the adipose tissue with a few interrupted sutures at the Scappa fascia. Closure of the Scappa fascia also ensures symmetry of skin closure. Blind closure of adipose tissue, in contrast to the Scappa fascia, is often met with annoying bleeding.

Skin is most commonly closed with monocryl suture (size U.S.P 3/O) placed in the subcuticular layer of the skin.

Maylard Incision

Dr Alfred Earnest Maylard, a surgeon at Victoria Infirmary, Glasgow, during the same era as Dr Pfannenstiel shared the common experience of the ail of midline laparotomy. He commented that "any surgeon who has set himself the task of carefully investigating the results of his median abdominal incisions not less than eighteen months or two years after their execution, cannot fail to have been impressed with the number of post-operative herniae that existed".

Dr Maylard further observed that herniation occurred in a median but not transverse abdominal incision in one of the patients he had operated on. In his investigation, evaluation, and deliberation of the patient's anatomy and physiology, he highlighted the rationale for a new transverse abdominal incision that bears his namesake today:

(i) The aponeurosis of external and internal oblique muscles that franks the anterior abdominal wall fuses densely at the lateral border of the rectus abdominis muscle to form the semilunaris. The fibers of the aponeurosis then split and traverse transversely and interdigitate with the longitudinally running fibers of the rectus abdominis. The transverse fibers form three to five dense bands that divide the long rectus abdominis muscle into segments. The three bands between the level of the umbilicus and the xiphisternum are the most prominent while the two below the umbilicus are more variable and may be absent.

(ii) The rectus abdominis has vast blood supply and an extensive lymphatic system, particularly at the anterolateral border where extensive anastomosis occurs between the deep inferior epigastric, internal mammary, and internal circumflex vessels. The vascular structures branch into capillaries toward and stop at the midline, without communication with the opposite side.

(iii) Transection of the rectus muscles does not weaken muscle contraction as the segmentation divides the contraction of the long rectus abdominis into units, and the excellent vasculolymphatic state results in good postoperative recovery.

In a publication in the *British Medical Journal* on October 5, 1907, Dr Maylard presented a series of 16 cases of transverse abdominal incisions. Of these, 12 (75%) were assessed to have perfect abdominal wall condition (no herniation) on follow up between 18 and 36 months after surgery. He concluded, in his own words, that "more permanently secure cicatrices result from transverse than vertical incisions".

The Maylard Incision has undergone several modifications, with some characteristics deserving special attention:

The original technique of the Maylard incision and its outcome

A semilunar incision is made in the skin just above the fold of Douglas halfway between the umbilicus and symphysis pubis, or 3.5 to 5 cm above the symphysis pubis. The transverse incision on the anterior sheath is curved upward slightly as it approaches the end laterally. There is no separation of the sheath from the recti abdominis muscle. The recti muscles are separated at the midline to gain access to the pelvis. Muscle division is done only when it is needed to achieve adequate incision aperture. The manner of muscle division is to deviate the direction of division obliquely upward at the lateral margin to maintain some intact muscle fibers. The severed end of the muscles is stitched to the rectus sheath to prevent retraction. At the completion of surgery, the incision is closed with deep mattress sutures.

Of the 41 cases studied in the original report, information was available for 13 cases of pelvic surgery: hysterectomy (7 cases), ovarian disease (4 cases), and ventrosuspension for uterine prolapse (2 cases). In all cases, both the right and left anterior sheaths were opened transversely, two had both recti abdominis completely divided, 6 had partial division, and five had no muscle division. Overall, three patients had hernia diagnosed during the study's follow up.

The modern Maylard incision

In current practice, the Maylard incision has been modified to become a planned procedure involving complete division of the rectus abdominis muscles and ligation of the inferior epigastric vessels.

A transverse skin incision about 2 to 3 cm above the symphysis pubis is made with a scalpel and extended at the midportion of the sheath using electrodiathermy. The sheath is opened through two small incisions at the sides of the midline. The upper and lower edge of the sheath are lifted up from the rectus muscles with two Kocher's forceps. The lateral extension of the incision, both subcutaneous adipose connective tissue and sheath is carried out with electrodiathermy toward the lateral border of the rectus muscle. At the lateral border of the rectus abdominis muscle, a long and curved Roberts artery clamp is inserted in a pointed up direction under the muscle and tracks along the undersurface of the muscle and above the transversalis fascia. The point of the clamp is brought out through the rectus muscle 1 cm lateral to the midline. The clamp is opened and a dry surgical gauze is grasped and pulled beneath the muscle from the midline to the lateral border of the muscle. The rectus abdominis is gently lifted up with a gauze sling and divided with long steady strokes of electrodiathermy (Figure 2.10). The inferior epigastric vessels will be seen with encircling fat toward the lateral margins of the muscle and can be grasped with a pair of artery forceps, cut, and ligated. The peritoneum is picked up with a pair of forceps and incised under direct vision. The incision is extended medially where the medial portions of the rectus muscle and the linea alba are divided. The peritoneum in the midline superiorly and inferiorly is sewn to the skin.

In the event of bleeding from the belly of the muscles that do not cease spontaneously, a large mattress suture can be used to incorporate the bleeding area. The suture should include the entire layers of the fascia, muscle, and peritoneum. Attention is needed to ensure that while the suture is tied firmly to stop the bleeding, it does not strangulate the muscle.

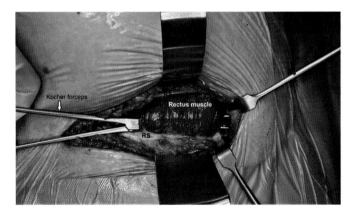

Figure 2.10 ■ A sketch illustrating the division of the rectus muscle in a Maylard incision.

Joel-Cohen Incision

In the earlier years of introducing the Joel-Cohen incision, many gynecologists practiced it as a modified version of the Pfannenstiel incision, contrary to Dr Sidney Joel-Cohen's vehement emphasis against it. The South African-born physician developed his technique of abdominal opening for gynecological surgery in 1954 to reduce surgical time, particularly for the cesarean section.

The original Joel-Cohen incision

In his original description of the technique, Dr Joel-Cohen made a straight skin incision between his outstretched index finger and thumb at 1.5 inches (3.8 cm) below an imaginary line joining the anterior superior iliac spines. The incision was extended by cutting through the subcutaneous tissue in the midline for a width of 1 to 1.5 inches (2.5 to 3.8 cm) to reach the rectus sheath. An incision of similar length was made on the sheath, avoiding the direct incision of the midline. The index fingers are inserted between the edges of the sheath to open the sheath to the length of the skin incision by stretching in the craniocaudal direction. This same maneuver also bluntly widened the subcutaneous tissue to the extent of the skin incision. The index fingers were then placed between the right and left rectus abdominis muscles to pull them apart in a sideway direction along the line of incision without upward and downward movement. The exposed parietal peritoneum is held up in the midline by two forceps, incised, and then extended transversely with scissors to the extent of the skin incision. Four interrupted sutures were used to sew the peritoneum to the skin edges.

The anatomical and physiological basis of the Joel-Cohen incision

Dr Joel-Cohen's primary objective in developing a new abdominal incision technique was to reduce operation time rather than a concern with the integrity of surgical wounds. It is conceivable that time is saved through forceful blunt dissection using fingers compared to dissection of layers of tissue with scalpels or scissors.

Much of the anatomical and physiological basis of the incision was inferred instead of objectively investigated at the time of technical development. Nevertheless, several of its advantages can be explained with current knowledge of the anatomy and physiology of the abdominal wall and tissue response to surgery.

The funneling shape of the false pelvis, with a decreasing transverse diameter toward the inlet of the pelvis, dictates that a straight-line skin incision should be placed higher from the symphysis pubis than that of the Pfannenstiel incision to achieve an equivalent abdominal aperture of the incision. The level, in reference to the symphysis pubis, of the terminal ends of the upwardly curved semilunar Pfannenstiel incision and the direct distance between the terminal ends are, in fact, close to that of the Joel-Cohen incision.

Compared to the semilunar incisions of Pfannenstiel and Maylard, Joel-Cohen's straight-line incision inflicts lesser skin and subcutaneous tissue trauma. As the blunt dissection stretches tissues along the plane of least resistance, less trauma occurs compared to when a sharp dissection is done. The neurovascular vessels, being stretched instead of disrupted by direct cutting, suffer a lesser extent of discontinuity. The hemostatic response of blood vessels to stretching is in stark contrast to the brisk bleeding of direct severance.

Being an incision at a position of 3 to 4 cm above the symphysis, together with the deviation of a straight-line skin incision from the direction of Langer's lines in the lower abdominal wall, the Joel-Cohen incision is less appealing in aesthesia than a standard Pfannenstiel incision.

The modern Joel-Cohen incision

With the epidemic of central obesity in modern society, the thickness of adipose tissue has significantly increased the difficulty of blunt dissection and the anchoring of the peritoneum to the skin. Today, almost all gynecologic surgeons perform the incision with some degree of variation from the original technique according to the physique of the patient.

— Low skin incision, which is feasible when a large surgical field is unnecessary;
— Blunt dissection of subcutaneous tissue to the sheath before opening the sheath;
— Separation of the sheath in a craniocaudal direction;
— Blunt opening of the peritoneum;
— It has been widely adopted for the cesarean section instead of elective gynecological surgery. The tissue edema in response to the influence of pregnancy hormones makes the tissues yield to blunt dissection easily.

Summary of Characteristics of Laparotomy Incisions

The 10 most common characteristics of these three transverse abdominal incisions are summarized in the following table for simple reference:

Characteristic	Type of Incision			
	Midline	Pfannenstiel	Maylard	Joel-Cohen
Surgical skill	+	++	+++	++
Operation time	+	++	+++	+
Surgical field	+++	++	++	++
Blood loss	+	++	+++	+
Wound hematoma	+	++	++	+
Nerve injury	+/−	++	+++	+
Postsurgery pain	++	+	++	+
Wound dehiscence	+	+/−	+/−	+/−
Hernia formation	+	+/−	+/−	+/−
Good aesthesia	+/−	+++	++	++
Note: "+" indicates increase in magnitude				

Guiding Principles in Choosing an Abdominal Incision

My guiding principles on the choice of abdominal incision are: (1) anatomy and physiology basis, (2) surgical appropriateness, (3) patient's constitutional condition, (4) evidence-based experience, and (5) surgical etiquette and wound aesthesia.

Anatomy and Physiology Basis

A prerequisite condition for good recovery from surgery is surgical technique that inflicts anatomical and physiological disturbances to the least extent. Dr Maylard's opening remark when introducing his new abdominal incision technique is a piece of sound advice: "If any result of our work is really and permanently successful, it must be because, in the execution of our object, we conform to Nature's laws, and do nothing that hinders her recuperative efforts in effecting what is her sole prerogative."

Structural disruption from surgical incision includes all compositions of the abdominal wall from skin, adipose tissue, and fascia to vascular, lymphatic, and neural tissues. In skin incision, as the transversely running Langer's lines assume a course in an infero-medial direction in the lower abdomen, a semilunar skin incision with the terminal parts curved upward would follow the direction of these lines more closely than a straight-line transverse incision.

Severance is the nature of surgery in order to access structures below the skin, but it should be kept to the least extent. On this point, Dr Maylard's advice again carries an important message. After an extensive deliberation, justification, and demonstration of the feasibility of severing the rectus abdominis muscle, he recommended that the rectus muscles should not be transected if separation of the muscles alone is adequate and, if transection of the muscle is necessary, the lateral muscle fibers should be spared. A complete transection of the rectus abdominis muscle is associated with cutting and ligating the inferior epigastric vessels. This procedure carries a risk of compromising collateral blood circulation to the lower limb.

Anatomical consideration also highlights that some surgeries carry a higher risk than others of injuring adjacent structures unintentionally. For example, compared to an incision limited to the midportion of the lower abdomen or a midline incision, a transverse incision extending laterally close to the anterior superior iliac spines has a higher risk of injuring the lateral femoral nerve and the iliohypogastric nerve.

The physiological process of wound healing has a paramount influence on the integrity and tensile strength of the wound and the strength of the abdominal wall in the long term. A midline incision where the vascular circulation is relatively lower and yet subject to strong lateral pulls from the abdominal muscles is weaker in tensile strength and has a high chance of hernia formation. In transverse incision, the aponeurosis is open in parallel to the fibrous fibers. The action of muscle contraction has little or no pulling force on the wound. Together with good vascular circulation, the integrity of the wound is good and thus heals better. Hernia formation is rare, though Dr Maylard reported in his study that herniation occurred in the midline of the transverse incision that he had performed on some of his patients.

Based on this principle, a transverse incision is preferred to a midline incision. Of the various types of transverse incision, the Pfannenstiel incision or Joel-Cohen incision is preferred to the Maylard incision. Dr Monroe Kerr, a contemporary of Dr Maylard in Glasgow, popularized the Pfannenstiel incision instead of the Maylard incision.

Surgical Appropriateness

Laparotomy incision opens the gate to the intra-abdominal or pelvic organs of the intended surgery. It follows that the gate must be appropriately placed and of sufficient dimension for the actual surgery. For surgery confined to the central pelvis, such as a total abdominal hysterectomy, when the diseased structure does not extend into the mid cavity of the abdomen, a transverse incision laparotomy is appropriate. For conditions that involve surgery in the upper part of the abdomen, a midline incision is a necessity.

To gain adequate access to the lateral pelvic side wall, a transverse incision with a rectus abdominis muscle transection may be necessary.

Patient's Constitutional Condition

Several characteristics of the patient's constitution have a significant impact on the choice of laparotomy incision.

— Nutritional, metabolic, and immune status, such as poorly controlled diabetes mellitus, malnutrition, long-term immunosuppressive therapy, or immunocompromise from a concurrent illness, prolong the process of wound healing and carry high risk of infection. Complications such as wound dehiscence and delayed healing or hernia formation in later phases may occur.

— Coexisting illnesses such as cancer or their related therapeutic medications such as anticoagulation are known to affect blood loss and wound hematoma formation. The presence of severe anemia will influence the patient's tolerance of blood loss. Chronic circulatory insufficiency and arteriosclerosis may be further compromised by certain incisions more than others.

— The patient's physique plays a role. Severe obesity with a generalized thick abdominal adipose tissue layer or a large pendulous abdomen is a challenge for all types of incision and may render some incisions more appropriate than others.

— Prior surgeries and outcome of wound healing play an important part in the decision of incision.

Evidence-based Experience

In the presence of multiple options, decisions on the type of laparotomy incision to use should be based on high quality clinical evidence. The best evidence through randomized controlled trials has never been conducted to investigate differences in the merits between midline and transverse abdominal incisions. Historical reports have indicated lower incidences of hernia formation in transverse than midline incisions. Differences in other outcomes such as chronic wound pain have yet to be investigated.

There is no randomized controlled trial evaluating the difference between the Pfannenstiel and Joel-Cohen incisions in total abdominal hysterectomy. Randomized controlled trials that compared these incisions for cesarean section reported favorable short-term outcomes for the Joel-Cohen incision in terms of operative time, blood loss, immediate postoperative pain and analgesia requirement, febrile illnesses, and length of hospital stay.

Surgical Etiquette and Wound Aesthesia

Etiquette of surgery refers to the less well-defined aspects of surgery which, nonetheless, can significantly violate Nature's law of anatomy and physiology. For example, in a seemingly uneventful hysterectomy, excessive electrocauterization to secure hemostasis can devitalize tissues and result in delayed tissue healing and an increased risk of surgical wound infection due to compromised immunity from disrupted blood circulation to the tissue. Unrefined surgical conduct, including forceful retraction on the wound and other organs, are often reflected in raised incidences of injuries to tissues and organs adjacent to the organ that the surgery is targeting, increased blood loss and need for replacement of blood or blood products to sustain adequate vascular circulation, impaired incision wound recovery, and increased peri-opeartive pain.

In this aspect, a finely conducted surgery is a display of skillful mastery of craft. I would prefer the Pfannenstiel incision to the Joel-Cohen incision.

Patient-centered outcome such as peri-operative experience and long-term wound pain and aesthesia of surgical wound is as important as objective surgical outcome. While high quality evidence is not available for the comparison of abdominal incisions, a well-healed and well concealed Pfannenstiel incision is more likely to appease the eyes.

References

Charoenkwan K, Iheozor-Ejiofor Z, Rerkasem K, *et al.* (2017) Scalpel versus electrosurgery for abdominal incisions. *Cochrane Database Syst Rev* 6(6): CD005987. doi: 10.1002/14651858. CD005987.pub2.

Deerenberg EB, Harlaar JJ, Steyerberg EW, *et al.* (2010) Review of advantages of Joel-Cohen surgical abdominal incision in caesarean section: A basic science perspective. *Med J Malaysia* 65(3): 204–208.

Mahendru R, Malik S, Mittal A, *et al.* (2011) Minilaparotomy hysterectomy: A worthwhile alternative. *J Obstet Gynaecol Res* 37(4): 305–312. doi: 10.1111/j.1447-0756.2010.01348.x. Epub 2011 Jan 5.

Mioton LM, Dumanian GA. (2018) Theoretic and evidence-based laparotomy closure with sutures and meshes. *Plast Reconstr Surg* 142(3 Suppl): 117S–124S. doi: 10.1097/PRS.0000000000004868.

Nygaard IE, Squatrito RC. (1996) Abdominal incisions from creation to closure. *Obstet Gynecol Surv* 51(7): 429–436. doi: 10.1097/00006254-199607000-00022.

Olofsson P. (2015) Opening of the abdomen ad modum Joel Cohen, Joel-Cohen, Joel Joel-Cohen, or just Cohen? *Acta Obstet Gynecol Scand* 94(2): 224–225. doi: 10.1111/aogs.12552. Epub 2014 Dec 30.

Olyaeemanesh A, Bavandpour E, Mobinizadeh M, *et al.* (2017) Comparison of the Joel-Cohen-based technique and the transverse Pfannenstiel for caesarean section for safety and effectiveness: A systematic review and meta-analysis. *Med J Islam Repub Iran* 31: 54. doi: 10.14196/mjiri.31.54.

Ortiz Molina E, Díaz de la Noval B, Rodríguez Suárez MJ, *et al.* (2020) Maylard's incision: How to make an easy incision for complex pelvic abdominal surgery. *Int J Gynecol Cancer* **30**(1): 154–155. doi: 10.1136/ijgc-2019-000876. Epub 2019 Oct 23.

Ramshorst GH, Kleinrensink GJ, Jeekel J, *et al.* (2015) Small bites versus large bites for closure of abdominal midline incisions (STITCH): A double-blind, multicentre, randomised controlled trial. *Lancet* **386**(10000): 1254–1260. doi: 10.1016/S0140-6736(15)60459-7. Epub 2015 Jul 15.

van Rooijen MMJ, Lange JF. (2018) Preventing incisional hernia: Closing the midline laparotomy. *Tech Coloproctol* **22**(8): 623–625. doi: 10.1007/s10151-018-1833-y. Epub 2018 Aug 9. PMID: 30094713; PMCID: PMC6154121.

Tay SK, Bromwich N. (1998) Outcome of hysterectomy for pelvic pain in premenopausal women. *Aust N Z J Obstet Gynaecol* **38**(1): 72–76. doi: 10.1111/j.1479-828x.1998.tb02963.x. PMID: 9521396.

3

Anatomy of Pelvic Structures Relevant to Hysterectomy

Introduction

By nature, hysterectomy or extirpation of the uterus disrupts the anatomical arrangement of the pelvic visceral ligaments and vasculolymphatic and neural structures. The responsibility of a gynecologist includes not only removing a diseased uterus with the patient's acceptance of the consequential loss of uterine functions, but also not compromising the functions of the remaining pelvic organs and structures. It goes beyond the surgeon's mere cognizance of the principles of anatomy and physiology. He or she must be equipped with absolute knowledge of the anatomical details of the pelvis: the appearance and location of the organs and structures as well as the spatial relationships between them. The surgeon is further challenged by the distortion of anatomical details from disease processes for which the hysterectomy is being undertaken.

This chapter aims to describe the details of pelvic anatomy that are relevant to hysterectomy for benign conditions. It provides the basis for the surgical steps of hysterectomy, with or without excision of the appendages. It also highlights the surgical approach to prevent inadvertent injuries to adjacent organs and structures, as well as to mitigate risk of untoward consequences that may manifest only a long time after hysterectomy.

The Uterus

The uterus occupies the central position of the pelvis (Figure 3.1). The lower portion of the uterus is connected to the vagina via the cervical attachment to the fornix of the vagina. It is attached to the urinary bladder anteriorly and rectum posteriorly. The upper

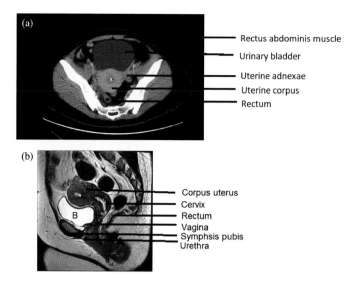

Figure 3.1 ■ Anatomical relationship of the pelvic viscera. (a) Computerized tomography image of the mid pelvis in coronal view and (b) magnetic resonance imaging of the pelvis in the sagittal plane.

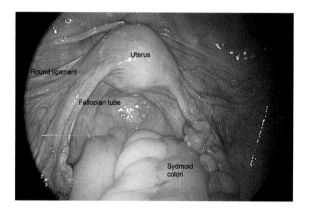

Figure 3.2 ■ A surgical photograph of the pelvic structures.

portion of the uterus is connected to the Fallopian tubes at the cornua points. The round ligaments are attached to the lateral borders of the uterine fundus immediately anterior and inferior to the Fallopian tubes.

Ovarian ligaments attach the ovaries to the uterus posterior and inferior to the Fallopian tubes (Figure 3.2). The Fallopian tube and ovary on each side are collectively referred to as the adnexa (pleura of adnexum in Latin) or appendage of the uterus. In gynecology, adnexae is the collective term for the right and left adnexa.

The uterus is anatomically divided into three parts (Figure 3.3):

(a) The cervix extends from the external os seen in the vagina to the internal os within the abdominal cavity. The level of the pelvic diaphragm divides the cervix to intravaginal and supravaginal portions.

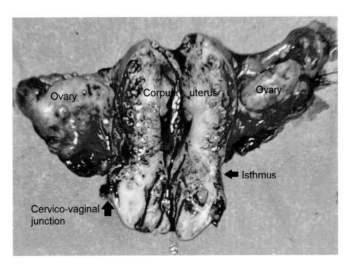

Figure 3.3 ■ A surgical photograph showing different parts of the uterus in a cut-open specimen in the sagittal plane.

The cervix is a fibromuscular structure with a predominance of fibrous tissue. The exact dimension of the cervix varies according to the status of circulating serum levels of estrogen and progesterone, and experience of parturition.

(b) The uterine isthmus is an arbitrary part where the cervix meets the body of the uterus. The isthmus marks the point where the fibromuscular structure of the cervix changes to become predominantly muscular tissue of the body of uterus. The level of the isthmus corresponds to the position of the vesicouterine fold of the anterior peritoneum immediately above the level of isthmus, the uterine artery divides into ascending and descending branches at the lateral borders of the uterus.

(c) The uterine corpus is the main part or the body of the uterus. In adult women, its dimension shows great variability depending on parity and diseases that Call for hysterectomy. It is a thick muscular structure with the muscle fibers arranged in three distinct layers of different orientation. The muscular layer of the uterus is called myometrium. The surface of the myometrium in the uterine cavity is lined by endometrium and the outer serosal border is known as perimetrium.

Uterine Fascia and Folds

Uterine Fascia

Pelvic fascia surrounding the uterus is an integral part of the parametrium. It is a layer of loose lymphovascular fatty tissue. Anterior to the abdominal portion of the cervix, it separates the cervix from the urinary bladder. Posteriorly, the fascia is franked by the uterosacral ligaments and provides a loose plane between the cervix and the rectum.

The fascia at the lateral borders of the uterus extends from the insertion of the Fallopian tubes to the pelvic floor, supporting the ureters, nerves, and lymphovascular structures.

Uterovesical Fold

The uterovesical fold is a distinct peritoneal fold formed by reflection of the anterior parietal peritoneum from the urinary bladder over loose cervical fascia to fuse with the tightly bound perimetrium of the uterus (Figure 3.4).

Insicion of the fold enters the vesicocervical space of loose fatty connective tissues. This is an important step in total hysterectomy and in lower segment cesarean section.

Rectouterine fold

Pelvic peritoneum between the uterosacral ligaments extends from the rectum over the posterior fornix of the vagina to fuse with the perimetrium of the uterus (Figure 3.2). The peritoneal reflection forms the rectouterine fold.

This fold covers the adipose connective tissue of the posterior parametrium and is the site of incision to enter the rectouterine space during hysterectomy and to access the rectovaginal septum for excision of deep infiltrative endometriosis.

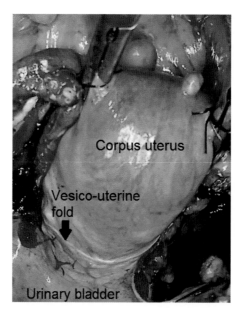

Figure 3.4 ■ A surgical photograph showing the vesicouterine fold of the peritoneum.

The Ligaments

Surgical anatomy illustrates six distinct uterine ligaments: broad ligaments, round ligaments, infundibulopelvic ligaments, uterosacral ligaments, cardinal ligaments, and vesicouterine ligaments. Of these, only the paired round ligaments and uterosacral ligaments are true ligaments in structure. The ligament nature of cardinal ligaments and vesicouterine ligaments are being disputed. Broad ligaments and infundibulopelvic ligaments are peritoneal folds.

Broad Ligaments

Broad ligaments are the mesentery attachments of the pelvic reproductive organs. Structurally, they are formed by the lateromedial extension of parietal peritoneum from the two pelvic sidewalls. The lateral portion of the broad ligament wraps round the uterine portion of the round ligament anteriorly (Figure 3.5). Lateroposteriorly, the portion of broad ligament that wraps round the infundibulum, the hylum portion (but not the cortex portion) of the ovary, and the suspensory ligament of the ovary are known as the mesovarium. The portion that wraps and attaches the Fallopian tube to the ovary in a curtain-like sheath is known as the mesosalpinx (Figure 3.6). The medial portion where

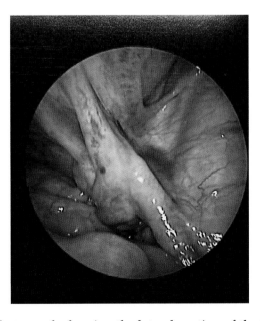

Figure 3.5 ■ A surgical photograph showing the lateral portion of the broad ligament wrapping the round ligament and infundibulopelvic ligament.

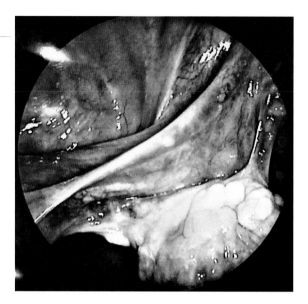

Figure 3.6 ■ A surgical photograph showing the mesosalpinx.

the right and left broad ligaments meet and densely adhere to the body of the uterus is known as the mesometrium, which forms the serous layer or perimetrium of the uterus. The anterior parietal peritoneum extends over the dorm of the urinary bladder and anterior uterine fascia to join the lower border of the perimetrium. The demarcation of this junction is distinct because of the loose fascia anterior to the cervix and tight adherence of the perimetrium.

Broad ligaments have no significant contribution to ligamental support but carry the vascular, lymphatic, and neural supply of reproductive organs. They also separate these organs from ureters. During hysterectomy, after division of the round ligament, the anterior and posterior leaf of the broad ligament can be separated easily to expose the ureter and vasculoneural structures of the pelvic sidewalls (Figure 3.7). Identification and lateral dissection of the ureters are important surgical maneuvers that safeguard them from injuries (Figure 3.8). Identifying the anterior division of the internal iliac artery allows the uterine artery to be isolated at its origin for ligation to control bleeding (Figure 3.9).

Round Ligaments

These paired structures are embryological remnants of gubernaculum. During embryo development, gubernaculum is attached to the lower pole of the gonad. The shrinking of gubernaculum is responsible for the migration of the gonad from a level at T10 to either the scrotum in males or a point at the mid-level of the pelvis in females. In the absence of androgens in the female embryo, the shrinking of gubernaculum is limited and the migration of the ovary stops in the pelvis. The remaining course of the gubernaculum forms the

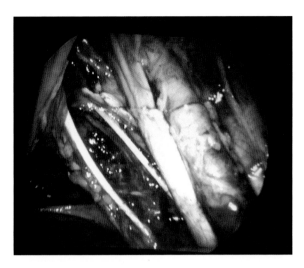

Figure 3.7 ■ A surgical photograph showing the vascular and neural structures exposed by opening the broad ligament space.

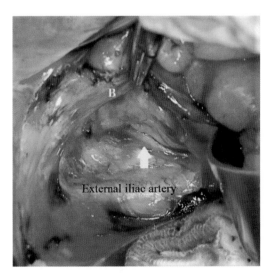

Figure 3.8 ■ A surgical photograph showing the relationship of ureter to infundibulopelvic ligament.

true ovarian ligament which attaches the ovary to the posterosuperior part of the uterus. The distal portion of the gubernaculum forms the round ligament which leaves the uterus and courses laterally to enter the internal ring of the inguinal canal and terminates in the labia majora, which corresponds to embryological equivalence of the scrotum in males.

Of surgical importance, round ligaments on the uterine end are closely related to the Fallopian tubes as they are located immediately anterior and inferior to the tubes. From the uterine insertion, these two structures take a divergent course. The Fallopian tubes are seen to course posterolaterally while round ligaments course anterolaterally (Figure 3.10).

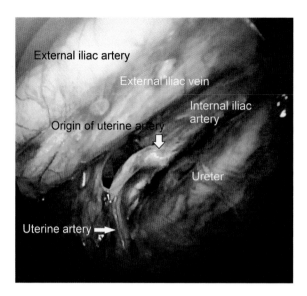

Figure 3.9 ■ A surgical photograph showing the origin of the uterine artery on the internal iliac artery.

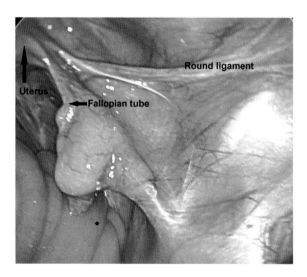

Figure 3.10 ■ A surgical photograph showing the anatomical position of the round ligament.

Inferiorly, round ligaments are attached to the superior part of the broad ligaments. Toward the uterine end of the round ligament, a branch of the ovarian artery known as Sampson's artery traverses inferiorly in parallel to and provides blood supply to the round ligament (Figure 3.11). Clamping and ligation of the round ligament during hysterectomy should include Sampson's artery to prevent bleeding.

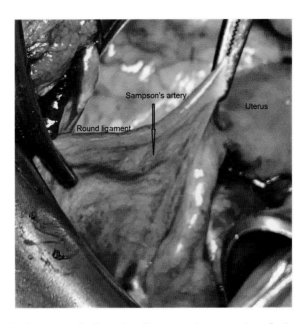

Figure 3.11 ■ A surgical photograph showing Sampson's artery in relation to the round ligament.

Infundibulopelvic Ligaments

The infundibulopelvic ligaments are paired structures that are also known as the suspensory ligament of the ovaries. They span from the infundibulum of the right and left ovaries to the pelvic sidewalls craniolaterally. The lateral ends of the ligaments cross the external iliac arteries and veins. The ureters, which cross the bifurcation of the common iliac arteries, are closely related to the inferior aspect of these ligaments (Figure 3.12). Clamping, ligation, and division of infundibulopelvic ligaments impose a risk of injuring ureters.

The infundibulopelvic ligament consists of peritoneum wrapping the ovarian blood and lymphatic vessels and nerve fibers. It is not a true ligament by anatomical structure as it suspends rather than supports the ovary.

Ovarian Ligaments

These are parts of remnant embryological gubernaculum distal to the ovaries. They anchor the ovaries to the lateroposterior surface of the uterus (Figure 3.13).

Uterosacral Ligaments

The paired uterosacral ligaments are fan-like structures extending from the sacrum to the cervix. At the sacral end, the ligament is attached with a broad base of approximately

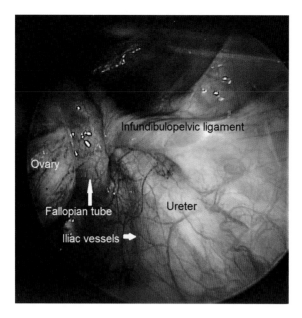

Figure 3.12 ■ A surgical photograph showing the position of the ureter in relation to the iliac artery and infundibulopelvic ligament.

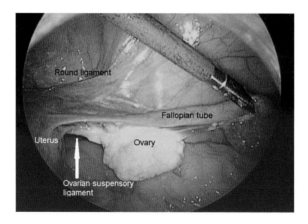

Figure 3.13 ■ A surgical photograph showing the ovarian suspensory ligament.

5 cm over the first three sacral vertebrae. The ligament tapers to a size of 2 cm at the insertion to the cervix. The attachment spans from the level of the internal os of the cervix to the superior portion of the vagina (Figure 3.14).

As the ureters course from the pelvic brim toward the cervix, they become increasingly closer to the anterior margin of the uterosacral ligament. At the point of cervical attachment, the ureters are 1 cm away from the uterosacral ligament (Figure 3.15). At the inferior margin of the ligaments, the middle rectal arteries are located at the middle portion and superior gluteal veins at the sacral ends.

The location of the ureter at the cervical insertion of the uterosacral ligament is a site of high risk for ureteric injury. Division of this ligament during hysterectomy should

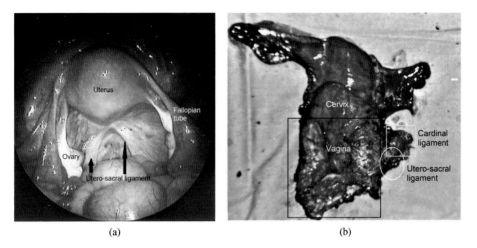

(a)   (b)

Figure 3.14 ■ Surgical photographs showing the uterosacral ligament.

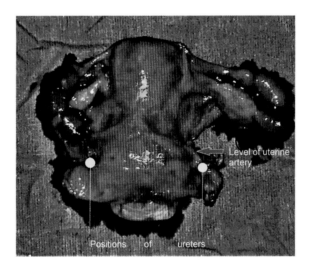

Figure 3.15 ■ A surgical photograph to demonstrate the position of the ureters at the level of the uterine cervix.

spare the vaginal portion to maintain good ligament support to the vagina. During closing of the vaginal vault, attachment of uterosacral ligaments to the vault or placating the two uterosacral ligaments together will mitigate the potential risk of vaginal vault prolapse or development of enterocoele later in the patient's life.

Cardinal Ligaments

Cardinal ligaments can be seen when the uterus is deviated to the contralateral side by traction. Previous terminology of these paired structures includes Mackenrodt's ligaments, named after the German gynecologist Dr A.K. Mackenrodt (1859–1925), lateral

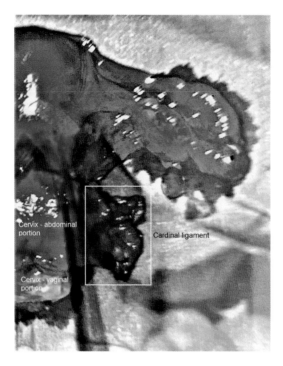

Figure 3.16 ■ A surgical photograph showing a cardinal ligament.

cervical ligaments, or transverse cervical ligaments. It forms the inferior border of the broad ligament at the level of the origin of the internal iliac artery and is superior to the pelvic diaphragm. It is attached to the cervix medially and extends laterally to attach to the obturator membrane of the pelvic side wall (Figure 3.16). At the cervical insertion, it is joined by the uterosacral ligament posteriorly and by the vesicouterine ligament anteriorly (Figure 3.17). Structurally, it is composed of connective tissues, muscle fibers, blood and lymphatic vessels, and nerve fibers. Cardinal ligaments, together with uterosacral and vesicouterine ligaments, stabilize the cervix. It collaborates with the pelvic floor musculature, rather than by itself, to form the main support of the uterus.

The uterine artery is located at the superior region and the veins are located at the inferior region of the cardinal ligaments. Medially and approximately 2 cm from the lateral border of the cervix, the ureter is located between the uterine artery anteriorly and the veins posteriorly (Figure 3.16). The inferior hypogastric nerve plexus is located toward the medial and inferior region of the cardinal ligament. These anatomical arrangements are important surgical considerations.

During a simple total hysterectomy, movement of cardinal ligaments by traction of the uterus in the direction of the median axis in relation to the trunk of the body moves the ureters away from the cervix, and cardinal ligaments are divided close to the border of the cervix. These maneuvers reduce the risk of ureteric injuries. For hysterectomy that requires excision of more than 2 cm of the upper vagina, further resection of the superior portion of the cardinal ligament over the ureter, the so-called roof of the ureteric tunnel,

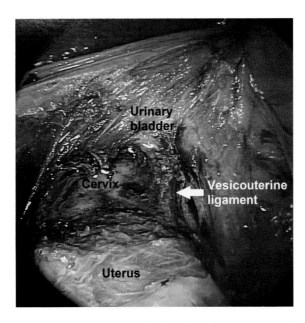

Figure 3.17 ■ A surgical photograph showing the vesicouterine ligaments.

is necessary to increase ureteric mobility in order to dissect the bladder from the upper vagina.

The deleterious impact of division of these ligaments supporting the vaginal vault and vagina has been dispelled.

Vesicouterine Ligaments

Vesicouterine ligaments are dense connective tissues that carry blood and lymphatic vessels and nerve fibers. They span from the cardinal ligaments to the bladder, marking the position of the ureterovesical junction and forming the lateral border of the vesicouterine space (Figure 3.17).

Dissection of vesicouterine ligaments are part of radical hysterectomy to ensure clearance of disseminated tumor cells from cervical or endometrial carcinoma. The dissection often disrupts the local neural network around the inferior hypogastric plexus with consequent denervation and functional alteration of the urinary bladder and rectum.

Blood Supplies

Uterine arteries and veins are the main blood supply of the uterus. The artery is a branch of anterior division of the internal iliac artery. From its origin, the artery travels horizontally

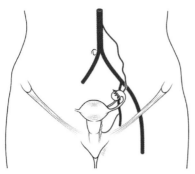
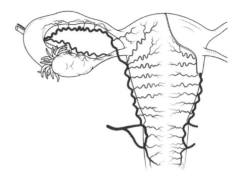

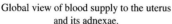

Global view of blood supply to the uterus and its adnexae.

Distribution of blood supply in the uterus and the anastomosis with ovarian vessels.

Figure 3.18 ■ Sketches to illustrate the distribution of blood supply to the uterus. Global view of blood supply to the uterus and its adnexae. Distribution of blood supply in the uterus and the anastomosis with ovarian vessels.

along the superior region of the cardinal ligament to the lateral border of the uterus. At the medial portion of the cardinal ligament, the artery crosses the ureter. The uterine vein in the inferior region of the cardinal ligament is posterior to the ureter. Ureters are at risk of injury at this location due to ligation of uterine vessels during hysterectomy.

At the level of and lateral to the uterine isthmus, the uterine artery divides into descending and ascending branches (Figure 3.18). The descending branch supplies the cervix and anastomoses with the vaginal artery. The ascending branch travels along the lateral border of the uterus and splits into five branches that penetrate the myometrium horizontally to supply the myometrium and endometrium. The fundal branch of the artery and veins anastomose with the ovarian vessels located between the Fallopian tube and suspensory ligament of the ovary. From here, a small artery branches off to supply the round ligament, known as the Sampson artery.

It is of clinical importance that the vast collateral blood supply of the uterus allows both uterine arteries to be ligated during management of uterine bleeding without compromising the vascular integrity to the uterus.

Nerve Supplies

The uterus is innervated by the autonomic nervous system. The sympathetic fibers from T10–12 and LI are carried in the hypogastric nerve which runs in parallel and approximately 3–4 cm below the ureter. The parasympathetic fibers from S2–4 are carried in the pelvic splanchnic nerve that runs along the inferior border of the cardinal ligament. Hypogastric and pelvic splanchnic nerves meet to form the inferior hypogastric nerve plexus, which gives out fibers to innervate the uterine corpus, cervix, and the vagina, as well as the urinary bladder.

A simple total hysterectomy has a low risk of jeopardizing the integrity of the inferior hypogastric plexus. On the other hand, extensive dissection of the parametrium around the cervix and upper vagina does frequently injure the plexus or main branches to the rectum or bladder, resulting in constipation and motor nerve impairment in the bladder with voiding disorders.

Lymphatic Drainage

Lymphatic draining of the uterus occurs through thin-walled lymphatic channels running along blood vessels. Anatomical and surgicopathological findings have established that almost 90% of lymphatic drainage finally follows two pathways known as the supraureteral and infraureteral paracervical pathways in the cardinal ligaments, where paracervical lymph nodes are located. The subsequent drainage follows the distribution of lymph nodes along the internal, external, and obturator vessels along the pelvic sidewalls. The fundal region of the uterus has the lymphatic drainage along the utero-ovarian vascular anastomosis to abdominal cavo-aortic lymph nodes.

Hysterectomy for benign conditions does not involve dissection of pelvic lymph nodes. There is no disruption of the overall lymphatic network of drainage in the pelvis or from the lower limbs.

The Parametrium

The parametrium encompasses the soft tissue structures surrounding the uterus and cervix. Anatomical orientation allows the parametrium to be described as the anterior, posterior, or right and left lateral parametrium.

Structures in the anterior parametrium include the fatty fascia between the urinary bladder and the cervix between the lateral pillars of the urinary bladder. The posterior parametrium includes the fibrous condensation extending from the lateral pelvic side walls at the location of the uterosacral ligaments to the upper vagina.

The lateral parametrium can be divided at the level of the cardinal ligament into the cranial and caudal portions. The cranial portion is the parametrium of the uterine corpus and consists of adipose tissue and the ascending uterine vessels. The uterine artery crosses the ureter at a point where the ureter enters the cardinal ligament. From this point onwards caudally, the lateral parametrium is also known as the paracervix, which spans between the bladder pillar and the uterosacral ligament at the lateral border of the uterus, in a fan-shape pattern, toward the pelvic side wall. It consists of the cardinal ligament, ureter medially approximately 1 cm lateral to the cervix, inferior hypogastric nerve plexus, deep uterine vein, and adipose tissue containing lymphatic vessels and lymph nodes.

Peritoneal Folds and Spaces

Anterior Peritoneal Folds

The thickening of the anterior parietal peritoneum at the lower part of the abdomen includes the median, medial, and lateral umbilical folds. The median fold contains the urachus while the right and left medial folds contain the obliterated umbilical arteries, which are the terminal branch of the anterior division of internal iliac arteries (Figure 3.19).

Peritoneal Spaces

a) The pouch of Douglas, named after Dr James Douglas (1675–1742), a Scottish anatomist, is also known as the rectovaginal pouch or cul-de-sac. It is the most caudal and, thus, most gravity-dependent part of the peritoneal cavity. It terminates at the reflection of the peritoneum of the posterior fornix of the vagina on to the rectum. It is related to the uterus and posterior fornix of the vagina anteriorly, rectum posteriorly, and broad ligaments laterally. Physiologically, it is lined by a thin film of peritoneal fluid and, sometimes, a small amount of retrograde menstrual blood. It is occupied by loops of small intestine and uterine corpus in cases of retroverted or retroflexed uterus. This is also the most common site of endometriosis, and the associated adhesion and fibrosis often result in loss of mobility of the uterus during hysterectomy.

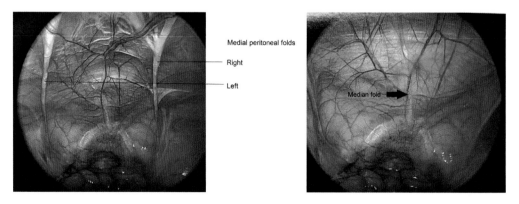

Figure 3.19 ■ Surgical photographs showing the median and medial umbilical folds.

b)   The vesicouterine pouch is a space of peritoneal cavity bounded by the urinary bladder anteriorly, the anterior surface of the uterus posteriorly, the broad ligament and round ligaments laterally, and the vesicouterine fold inferiorly is known as the vesicouterine space.

Deposits of endometriosis and intraperitoneal cancer are often found in the vesicouterine pouch. Incision of the pouch at the vesiouterine fold is the surgical method to access the cervix for a total hysterectomy and for incision of the uterus during lower segment cesarean section.

Retroperitoneal Spaces

Several retroperitoneal spaces are described for radical hysterectomy. During hysterectomy for benign conditions such as deep infiltrative endometriosis or for accessing the retroperitoneal vascular structures to secure hemostasis, knowledge of paravesical and pararectal spaces are important.

Paravesical Spaces

The right and left paravesical spaces are relatively avascular spaces of loose connective tissue between the pillars of the urinary bladder medially and the pelvic side walls laterally. These are related to the lateral umbilical fold superiorly, arcuate lines of the ilium anteriorly, the cardinal ligament posteriorly, and pubocervical fascia on the levator ani muscle inferiorly.

Pararectal Spaces

The avascular loose connective tissue spaces between the rectum medially and the pelvic side walls laterally are the right and left pararectal spaces. These are related to the broad ligament superiorly, the cardinal ligament anteriorly, the uterosacral ligament and rectum medially, and the levator ani muscle inferiorly.

Pelvic Floor Muscles

The levator ani muscles consist of puborectalis, pubococygeos, and iliococygeous parts and form the main support for the pelvic organs. The puborectalis muscles originate from the inferior aspect of the pubis symphysis and superior fascia of the pelvic diaphragm, looping around the vagina and neck of the urinary bladder to form the bladder sphincter for maintaining urinary continence. The pubococygeous muscle originates from the pubic rami and loops around the rectum to support it.

During hysterectomy for benign conditions, the limited dissection close to the cervix and vagina inflicts no injuries to the pelvic floor muscular structures and has no impact on the supportive function of the levator ani muscles to the urinary bladder or rectum.

References

Bajka M, Manestar M, Hug J, *et al.* (2004) Detailed anatomy of the abdomen and pelvis of the visible human female. *Clin Anat* **17**(3): 252–260. doi: 10.1002/ca.10215. Erratum in: Clin Anat. 2004 Jul;17(5):450.

Balgobin S, Jeppson PC, Wheeler T 2nd, *et al.* (2020) Standardized terminology of apical structures in the female pelvis based on a structured medical literature review. *Am J Obstet Gynecol* **222**(3): 204–218. doi: 10.1016/j.ajog.2019.11.1262. Epub 2019 Dec 2.

Buller JL, Thompson JR, Cundiff GW, *et al.* (2001) Uterosacral ligament: description of anatomic relationships to optimize surgical safety. *Obstet Gynecol* **97**: 873–879.

Cunha GR, Robboy SJ, Kurita T, *et al.* (2018) Development of the human female reproductive tract. *Differentiation* **103**: 46–65. doi: 10.1016/j.diff.2018.09.001. Epub 2018 Sep 6.

Dietrich CS 3rd, Gehrich A, Bakaya S. (2008) Surgical exposure and anatomy of the female pelvis. *Surg Clin North Am* **88**(2): 223–243, v. doi: 10.1016/j.suc.2008.01.003.

Gray's Anatomy. Chapter 5 Pelvis #1; pp 423–481.

Jiménez AM, Colomer AT. (2008) An update of anatomical references in total laparoscopic radical hysterectomy: from surgical anatomy to anatomical surgery. *J Minim Invasive Gynecol* **15**(1): 4–10. doi: 10.1016/j.jmig.2007.07.009.

Samaan A, Vu D, Haylen BT, *et al.* (2014) Cardinal ligament surgical anatomy: cardinal points at hysterectomy. *Int Urogynecol J* **25**(2): 189–195. doi: 10.1007/s00192-013-2248-y. Epub 2013 Oct 30.

4

Abdominal Hysterectomy Procedure

Introduction

The surgicotechnical details of hysterectomy vary greatly between surgeons and from patient to patient according to the pathological condition of the uterus and pelvis. Nonetheless, a step-by-step account of the process in a typical scenario will highlight the applications of anatomical knowledge and surgical principles to achieve a hysterectomy proficiently and safely. It also provides a basis on which variation and adaptation can be done according to individual operative conditions, as will be illustrated as I elaborate on some of my personal views.

This chapter describes the procedures for three types of hysterectomy: total hysterectomy, subtotal hysterectomy, and hysterectomy with bilateral salpingo-oophorectomy. Salpingectomy is not part of hysterectomy by definition. As the Fallopian tubes cease to serve a purpose after hysterectomy and are a potential source of hydrosalpinx and high-grade serous adenocarcinoma, they are recommended to be removed together with hysterectomy.

Urinary Bladder and Vaginal Preparation

After adequate anesthesia and blood circulatory access are established, the vulva and perineum are painted with antiseptics. Transurethral catheterization of the urinary bladder is done for continuous drainage. The vagina is painted with povidone iodine.

Abdominal Skin Preparation

On entering the old University College Hospital (UCH) building on Gower Street, London, and at the top of a short staircase, I never missed casting a glance on the large wall portrait of Dr Joseph Lister (1827–1912). Lister was a medical student and house surgeon at UCH. Later, he took the chair of Professor of Surgery at the University of Glasgow, Scotland. During his time, many patients who underwent successful surgery died in the postoperative period from "water fever", a term for sepsis then. He took interest in two important findings of the day: Semmelweiss demostrated the dramatic benefit of reducing maternal mortality from postpartum fever when medical staff washed their hands before attendance to women in labor, and Luis Pastor reported that microbes turned wine sour in 1865. He developed a hypothesis that microbes were responsible for postsurgical fever and mortality and advocated skin preparation with an antiseptic, carbolic acid, before surgery. His success in improving the safety of surgery laid the foundations for antiseptic practice in surgery today.

It is important to note that the most common microbes causing surgical wound sepsis at the lower part of the abdomen are skin commensals and anogenital bacteria. The sequence of wiping of antiseptic from the upper abdominal skin down to the upper thighs in a one-way direction would reduce mechanical transfer of anogenital bacteria to the abdominal skin. Chlorhexidine solution and povidone iodine are antiseptics most commonly employed for skin preparation. The exposed skin around the position of incision part of the skin is further covered with sterile surgical drapes.

Instrument Preparation

Experienced surgeons are versatile with general surgical instruments. Each surgeon works best with a familiar set of instruments and equipment suiting his or her dexterity and ergonomic considerations. As instruments are prepared and supplied by a third-party facility, the scrubbed-up nurse will check the instruments for accountability, but the surgeon has to ensure that his preferred instruments are available.

The key instruments in my hysterectomy set include:

Pedicle clamps

— Curved and straight Masterson clamps, 216 mm: Atraumatic locking forceps with serration and longitudinal grooves to prevent tissue slipping, good for vascular pedicles.
— Roberts artery forceps, 230 mm: Non-toothed locking tissue forceps with serration, suitable for thin pedicles with low risk of tissue slipping.

Dissecting scissors

— Curved Mayo scissors, 170 mm: Heavy dissection scissors for thick pedicles and fibrotic or scarred tissues.
— Curved Metzenbaum dissecting scissors, 180 mm: Light dissecting scissors for thin and soft tissue dissection.

Dissecting tissue forceps

— Bonney's dissecting forceps, 180 mm: Toothed tissue grasping forceps for handling the edge of thick tissues.
— Straight Debakey dissecting forceps, 200 mm and 243 mm: Light non-toothed tissue grasping forceps for handling thin and soft tissues, including holding bleeding vessels or tissues for electrocoagulation.
— Littlewood tissue forceps, 191 mm: Ringed and ratcheted tissue holding forceps that allow good grasping and retracting tissues (other than visceral tissues).
— Babcock forceps, 150 mm: Atraumatic forceps suitable for soft tissues that are easily damaged, such as the Fallopian tubes.

Retractors

— Deaver abdominal retractors — narrow retractor, 25 mm × 305 mm; broad retractor, 51 mm × 305 mm: Retraction of visceral structures to improve exposure of pelvic cavity and retroperitoneal spaces.
— Morris abdominal retractor, 70 × 40 mm: Retraction of the abdominal wall to improve surgical view.

Laparotomy Incision

A laparotomy incision is performed as described in the previous chapter.

Intra-abdominal Preparation

Exploration: once the peritoneal cavity is entered, a careful inspection and gentle palpation of vital organs of intra-abdominal and pelvic viscera are performed to take note of the pathology.

Preparing a clear access to the pelvis: The patient is placed on a slight Trendelenburg position (5 to 10 degrees) and intestinal loops placed and held in abdominal cavity with two wet surgical gauge packs. Self-retaining retractors are used to maintain optimal laparotomy aperture.

Preparation of the Uterus

For the ease of handling, the uterus is held with two curved Masterson clamps at the lateral borders to include the uterine ends of the Fallopian tubes, round ligaments and ovarian ligaments. The assistant surgeon is reminded that, for the entire hysterectomy procedure, these two clamps are the only ones that traction can be applied on manipulating the uterus.

Procedure Steps in Total Hysterectomy

Hysterectomy in Three Pedicles

During my residency training in London, I was taught to perform hysterectomy in three pedicles. The first pedicle grasped the round ligament, Fallopian tube, and ovarian ligament together. This detached the upper part of the uterus from its appendages. The second pedicle clamped the uterine blood vessels. The third clamp took the parametrium which included the uterosacral ligament, cardinal ligament, and vesicouterine ligament (Figure 4.1). Once the procedures were completed bilaterally, the uterus was then ready to be amputated from the vagina.

I was impressed by the proficiency of the procedure. I acquired the technique well and performed many hysterectomies in this manner over a number of years. Admittedly on reflection, the early course of acquiring the technique was a struggle for me because the clamps were necessarily large and heavy for the big pedicles and my hands were much smaller than those of the British gynecologists, who were generally a-foot-and-a-half taller than me.

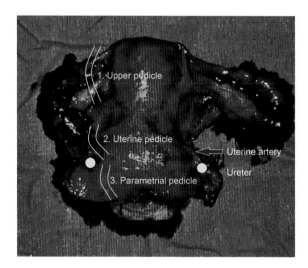

Figure 4.1 ■ Illustration of the position of the three pedicles in a total hysterectomy.

One day, I was called by a general surgeon who, during an anterior resection of the bowel found that the left uterine adnexa was involved by the disease and needed to be excised. He requested my assistance for him to do the salpingo-oophorectomy. He was very pleased on completion of the surgery, but I was impressed by his slow and elegant step-by-step basic anatomical dissection technique. Enlightened, I decided that hysterectomy would be physically less demanding and more graceful in terms of surgical etiquette if I do it according to individual anatomical parts. As I describe below, this technique will demonstrate well the anatomical principles of hysterectomy to my residents.

Hysterectomy by Individual Anatomical Parts

Division of round ligaments

The uterus is deviated medially to the contralateral side. The slight tension helps with the identification of the course of the round ligament. If necessary, further tension on the round ligament can be achieved by lifting the abdominal wall with a Morris retractor placed near the internal inguinal ring.

Two Roberts artery clamps, a centimeter apart, are used to grasp the round ligament at the midpoint between the uterus and the pelvic side wall. The grasped tissue should include the entire thickness of the round ligament and the Sampson artery running in parallel to and at the inferior border of the ligament (Figure 4.2). The round ligament and Sampson artery are divided perpendicularly between the clamps with electrodiathermy

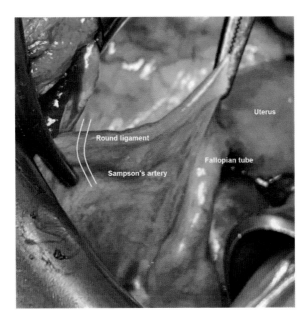

Figure 4.2 ■ A surgical photograph showing the clamping of the left round ligament, incorporating Sampson's artery.

coagulation or by a clean cut with Mayo scissors. This procedure opens the superior border of the broad ligament.

The lateral stumps of round ligament and Sampson artery are ligated with a Vicryl-O suture. The end of the suture is held with mosquito artery forceps.

The edge of the opened broad ligament is held with the Debakey forceps and the incision is extended anteriorly toward the isthmus of the uterus. A short extension of the broad ligament incision is done toward the pelvic brim, keeping the incision in parallel and a short distance lateral to the infundibulopelvic ligament.

Salpingectomy

The Fallopian tube is straightened with mild tension between the uterus and a pair of Babcock tissue forceps grasping the fimbrial end of the tube. The curtain-like mesosalpinx is seen outstretched, showing the ovarian vessels at the ovarian end of the curtain. Two or three branches of arteries are seen through the transparency of the mesosalpinx. They ascend perpendicularly to join the Fallopian tube vessels running in parallel and inferior to the length of Fallopian tube. The avascular portion of the mesosalpinx between the perpendicular arteries are incised, and the arteries clamped with artery forceps and divided and ligated with Vicryl-O sutures (Figure 4.3 shows the lines of incision in the mesosalpinx). The Fallopian tube is mobilized to the uterine end to be removed together with the uterus.

Identification of the ureter

Tracing the course of the ureter is not necessary in most cases of total hysterectomy. However, in cases where there is suspicion of deviation of its usual course from uterine pathology, such as huge leiomyoma or the presence of severe fibrosis in the

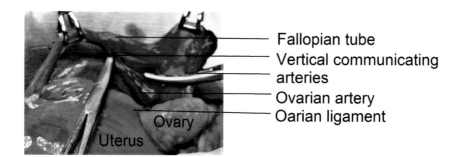

Figure 4.3 ■ A surgical photograph showing a salpingectomy. The vertical communicating arteries are identified and clamped, divided, and ligated to mobilize the Follopian tube up to its insertion point on the uterus.

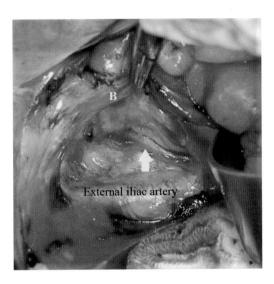

Figure 4.4 ■ A surgical photograph showing the ureter (yellow arrow) on the posterior leave of the broad ligament ("B"), immediately inferior to the infundibulopelvic ligament.

pelvis, it is critical to visually identify and lateralize the ureter to prevent its inadvertent injury.

From the incised broad ligament, the loose areolar tissue blunt dissection will expose the posterior leaf of the broad ligament. Gentle traction on an abdominal Deaver retractor is used to render the posterior broad ligament taut. The ureter with peristalsis can be seen 3 to 4 cm below the midportion of the infundibulopelvic ligament (Figure 4.4). If the ureter is not displayed by this maneuver, it can invariably be identified at the pelvic brim where it crosses the bifurcation of the common iliac artery.

The ureter is then lateralized from the broad ligament by gentle blunt dissection with the blade of a pair of right-angled artery forceps until it is seen to be close to the uterine artery at the point it enters the cardinal ligament.

The ovarian and utero-ovarian vessel pedicle

After mobilization of the Fallopian tube from the mesosalpinx, the utero-ovarian vessels are seen in a tortuous and engorged plexus in the broad ligament immediately superior to, and separated by a short distance from, the ovarian suspensory ligament (Figure 4.5). A small avascular window in the mesosalpinx can be identified between the complex of utero-ovarian blood vessels and ovarian ligament. The window is opened with the sharp tip of a closed right-angle artery forceps. The pedicle is clamped with two Roberts artery forceps, divided and transfixed using a Vicryl-O suture for secure hemostasis (Figure 4.5). The slender ovarian ligament is clapmed in Roberts forceps, divided and ligated with a Vicryl-0 suture.

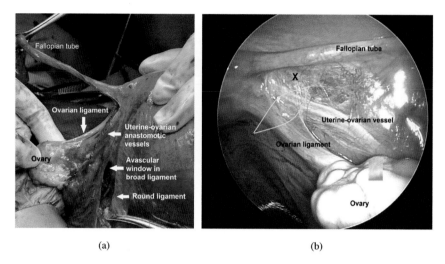

(a)   (b)

Figure 4.5 ■ Surgical photographs showing ligation of the ovarian ligament and utero-ovarian vessels in a single pedicle.

The uterine artery pedicle

The uterus is put under gentle traction and the vesicouterine fold of peritoneum at the midline is lifted upwards with a pair of tissue forceps and incised with Metzenbaum scissors. The peritoneal incision is extended at both directions to complete the incision on the anterior broad ligament (Figure 4.6). With the tip of the scissors slightly open and at a right angle to the peritoneal incision, the peritoneum is pushed downwards to expose a portion of the cervix. As the procedure approaches the lateral bladder pillars on the side of the cervix, bleeding can occur from the rich blood vessel structures. The reflection of peritoneum must be limited to the superficial layer of areolar tissues.

The areolar tissue at the upper parametrial border of the uterus is also pushed away gently to reduce the thickness of tissues to be taken in the uterine pedicle. Attention is needed at this position to avoid unnecessary bleeding from injury in the ascending branch of the uterine artery.

The position of the ureter in relation to the uterine artery at the border of uterus is checked. The ureter, if not visualised by lateralisation dissection earlier, can be palpated as a cord-like structure between the thumb and fingers.

A curved Masterson forceps is applied with the tips of the blades at the level of the uterine isthmus anteriorly and at the level immediately above the uterosacral ligament posteriorly, with the curved body of the forceps in an almost horizontal position. On closing the clamp slowly, the tip slips gently off the lateral border of the uterus and the body of the clamp grasps the uterine artery at the point where the vessels reach the uterus (Figure 4.7). The clamp is closed lightly and the ureter is palpated to confirm that it lies inferior and lateral to the clamp. The clamp is then tightened to complete the closure. A second clamp is applied similarly in parallel and medial to the first clamp,

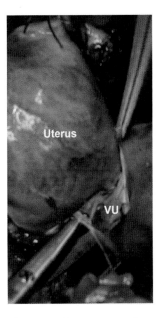

Figure 4.6 ■ A surgical photograph showing the opening the vesicouterine fold of the peritoneum.

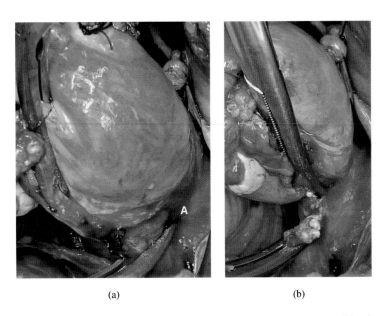

(a)   (b)

Figure 4.7 ■ Surgical photographs showing clamping (a) and dividing (b) of uterine vessels.

with a small gap in between the clamps for pedicle division using a sharp scalpel. Complete division of the pedicle is assured by freedom of the tip of the clamp from the uterus (Figure 4.7).

A curved needle Vicryl-O suture is used to ligate the pedicle. It is important to hold the clamp steadily without traction, twisting, or elevation to avoid pedicle slipping or avulsion and to avoid distortion in the position of the ureter.

Parametrium pedicle

Holding the uterus in a straight position under some tension, the vesicocervical space is further dissected to reflect the bladder down to the anterior vaginal fornix. The end of the cervix can be palpated between the surgeon's thumb and fingers placed anteroposteriorly around the cervix. The pouch of Douglas is inspected and rectal adhesion, to the posterior part of the cervix and uterus is released.

The parametrium pedicle in a simple total hysterectomy incorporates the uterosacral ligament, cardinal ligament, and paracervical tissues. This is secured with a straight Masterson clamp, which is applied close to the lateral border of the uterus and supravaginal cervix. Attention is needed to ensure that the clamp is medial to and does not incorporate the uterine pedicle (Figure 4.8). The tip of the clamp is checked to ensure that it has not incorporated part of the bladder. A long handle sharp scalpel is used to cut the clamped pedicle at the border of the uterus and cervix, keeping close to the side of the clamp. A Vicryl-O suture is used to transfix the pedicle. This pedicle is thicker than the other pedicles so far described. The position of the surgical knot should be placed at the midpoint of the pedicle to prevent part of the pedicle from slipping when the clamp is released.

Colpotomy

Urinary bladder is held with a right-angle bladder retractor to expose the cervix and vaginal fornix. Two Littlewood forceps are applied: one over the palpated lower bor-

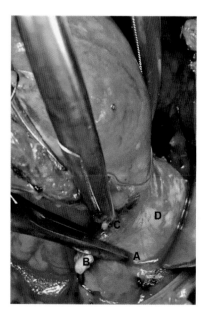

Figure 4.8 ■ A surgical photograph showing clamping of the parametrium pedicle: (A) Position at the border of the supravaginal cervix and clear from the bladder, (B) the stump of uterine vessels, (C) uterine stump of uterine vessels, and (D) the midline position over the cervix.

der of the cervix and one over the vaginal fornix. The two forceps are gently lifted upwards, keeping the tissue between them in horizontal position. Vagina is entered in a perpendicular stab incision with a sharp scalpel or by cutting electro-diathermy (Figures 4.9 A & B). The Littlewood forceps at the border of the cervix is repositioned to grasp directly onto the anterior lip of the cervix. Traction on the cervix exposes the entire cervix. Amputation of the vagina around the cervix is performed with a curved Mayo scissors or cutting electro-diathermy under direction vision. The uterus is thus removed completely.

The vaginal angles

The right and left corners of the vagina incision, or vaginal angles, are the position of anastomosis between the descending branch of uterine (cervical) artery and the ascending branch of vaginal artery. A figure-of-8 suture to each vaginal angle is the most reliable and secure management for these pedicles. A Roberts forceps is applied to the angle. The tip of the forceps is immediately inferior and medial to the pedicle of cardinal ligament. The forceps firmly grips the full thickness of the vaginal wall, including the mucosa layer (Figure 4.10A). With the bladder pushed away with a right-angle bladder retractor, the first loop of figure-of-8 (Vicryl-O) suture is inserted medially, ensuring that the suture includes the full thickness of vaginal wall and the peritoneum on the posterior edge of the vagina (Figure 4.10B). The second loop of the suture is placed immediately medial to the parametrium pedicle to occlude bleeding between these two pedicles (Figures 4.10 C & D). The end of the suture is held in position with a mosquito forceps.

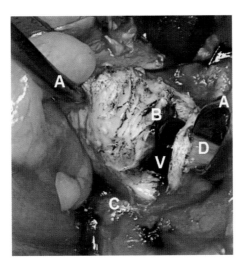

Figure 4.9A ■ A surgical photograph showing colpotomy with an incision into the anterior vaginal fornix. (A) Littlewood forceps to lift up the cervix; (B) anterior lip of the cervix; (C) stump of parametrium; (D) anterior vaginal wall; and (V) the lumen of vagina.

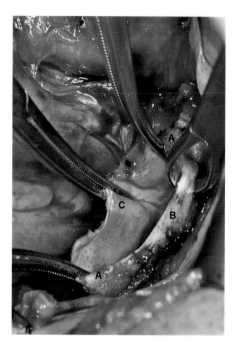

Figure 4.9B ■ A surgical photograph showing completed colpotomy.

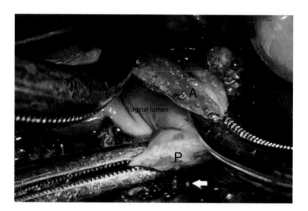

Figure 4.10A ■ a surgical photograph showing the vaginal angle on the right side. The anterior and posterior edge of vagina are marked with letters A and P respectively. Letter C indicates the parametrium pedicle.

Vaginal vault closure

Roberts forceps are applied at midpoint of anterior and posterior vaginal wall to ensure that the vaginal incision can be closed symmetrically (Figure 4.9B). The remaining portion of vaginal vault is closed with a continuous locking or interrupted horizontal mattress Vicryl-O suture. This suture begins immediately medial to the vaginal angle pedicle (Figures 4.10E, F & G).

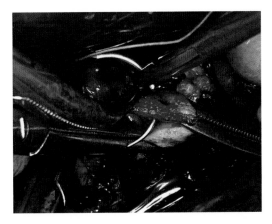

Figure 4.10B ■ A needle passed through the entire thickness of anterior edge of vagina.

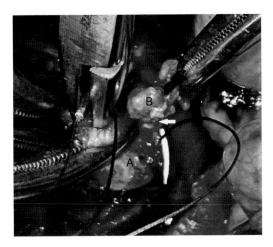

Figure 4.10C ■ The insertion of second loop of figure-of-8 immediately inferior and medial to parametrium pedicle. A = vaginal angle pedicle; B = parametrium pedicle held laterally with a artery forceps.

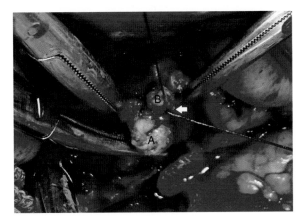

Figure 4.10D ■ Completion of figure-of-8 suture obliterating the death space between vaginal angle an parametrium pedicles marked by the solid white arrow.

Procedure Steps in Subtotal Hysterectomy

For subtotal hysterectomy. treatment of upper uterine pedicles follows the same steps as in total hysterectomy. The remaining steps are below:

Amputation of the corpus uterus

An incision across the uterine isthmus at the level immediately above the uterine pedicles is made with a cutting electro-diathermy pen. The incision is deepened until the upper

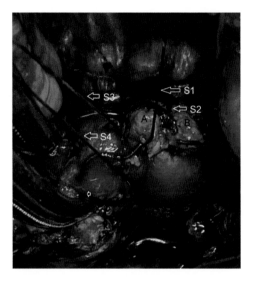

Figure 4.10E ■ The initial stitch of continuous locking suture placed imeediately medial to the vaginal angle pedicle. S1= holding suture of vaginal angle; S2 suture on parametrium pedicle; S3 and S4 are the two ends of the first stitch of continuous suture.

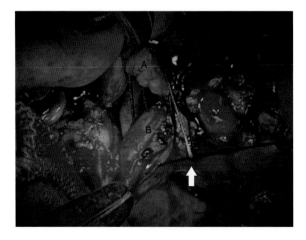

Figure 4.10F ■ Running continuous locking suture across the vaginal vault.

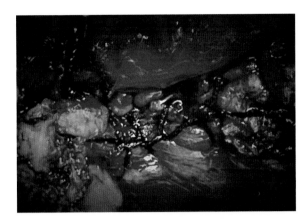

Figure 4.10G ■ Completed closure of vaginal vault.

end of the endocervical canal is entered. The incision is extended circumferentially round the posterior part of the cervix. The uterine corpus is thus removed (Figure 4.11).

Reversed conization of the cervix

Littlewood forceps are applied to the midpoint of the cut edge of the cervix anteriorly and posteriorly. A circular incision over the cervical stroma is made with an electrodiathermy pen, leaving a rim of cervix approximately 5-mm in thickness (Figure 4.12). The circular incision is extended in a conical direction, tapering toward the external os of the cervix. A cone of cervical stroma is thus removed.

This step is often omitted by many gynecologists, particularly in laparoscopic subtotal hysterectomy. Reversed conization of the cervix reduces the volume of cervical stroma for the following three good reasons:

(i)   To prevent menstruation after subtotal hysterectomy: Menstruating endometrium may extend beyond the level of amputation of the uterine corpus. In premenopausal women with intact ovarian function, cyclic menstruation may continue after a subtotal hysterectomy. This would be disappointing to women who elect for hysterectomy to terminate menstruation permanently.

(ii)   To reduce excessive cervical secretion after subtotal hysterectomy: Since the 1930s, total hysterectomy has been recommended in place of subtotal hysterectomy in the English-speaking world to prevent excessive vaginal discharge from the cervix and to reduce risk of cervical carcinoma. These intentions are, to a great extent, achieved by reducing the volume of cervical stroma glands in subtotal hysterectomy.

(iii) To minimize risk of endocervical carcinoma of the cervix: The incidence of cervical cancer in industrialized countries has been significantly reduced by regular screening programs over the last few decades. The benefit of screening is largely in preventing ectocervical carcinoma. Endocervical carcinoma, and adenocarcinoma in particular,

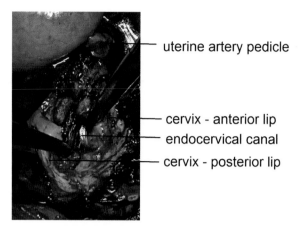

uterine artery pedicle

cervix - anterior lip
endocervical canal
cervix - posterior lip

Figure 4.11 ■ A surgical photograph showing the stump of cervix at subtotal hysterectomy.

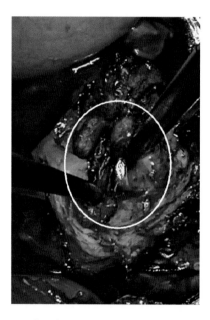

Figure 4.12 ■ A surgical photograph where the white-lined circle marks the position of the case of cone biopsy.

has dominated cervical cancer in recent years in these countries. Reversed conization of the cervix reduces both the glandular tissue and squamous transformation zone of the cervix within the endocervical canal. Thus, tissues are reduced from which cervical carcinoma arises.

Closure of the cervix

Once hemostasis on the cervix is ensured, the abdominal part of the cervix is closed with a Vicryl-O suture in figure-of-8 stitches.

Procedure Steps in Hysterectomy with Salpingo-Oophorectomy

Infundibulopelvic pedicle

After securing the round ligament pedicle, the infundibulopelvic ligament is put under slight tension by deviating the uterus anteriorly toward the midline. The broad ligament is opened from the superior border and the ureter is lateralized to a clear distance from the infundibulopelvic ligament (Figure 4.4). The ovary is mobilized from the ovarian fossa and inspected along the infundibulopelvic ligament for any accessary ovarian tissues. A window is made in the posterior leaf of the broad ligament immediately below the infundibulopelvic ligament. The skeletonized infundibulopelvic ligament is then clamped by two curved Masterson forceps (Figure 4.13).

Attention is called here to ensure that no ovarian tissue is included in the clamps to avoid residual ovarian syndrome. It is also important to avoid placing the clamps too near to the pelvic end of the ligament. The ureter converges toward the infundibulopelvic ligament in its course toward the iliac vessels laterally and is prone to iatrogenic injury.

The infundibulopelvic ligament is divided between the clamps using a sharp scalpel or scissors and the stumps are ligated. It is customary to put two ligatures on the proximal stump as bleeding from the ovarian artery, which branches directly from the descending aorta, is potentially catastrophic.

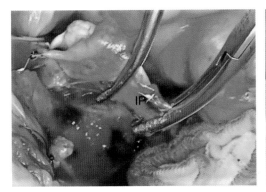 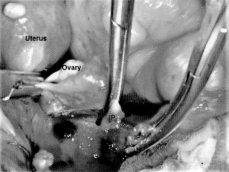

Figure 4.13 ■ A surgical photograph showing the clamping of the infundibulopelvic ligament in a case of hysterectomy with salpingo-oophorectomy.

The incision on the posterior leaf of the broad ligament below the ovarian and Fallopian tube is extended to the lateral border of the uterus immediately above the insertion of the uterosacral ligament. Preparation for the uterine pedicle and the rest of the hysterectomy procedure is the same as that described earlier for total hysterectomy.

Preparation for closure of the abdomen
Hemostasis confirmation

After removal of visible blood, the pelvic cavity is irrigated with warm sterile water to detect and stop any bleeding from the pedicles or edge of the broad ligament, or in the vesicocervical space.

Insertion of the pelvic drainage tube

This is rarely required in hysterectomy. However, in cases with a wide area of raw surface from extensive dissection and adhesiolysis, a surgical drain may be inserted for closed system continuous draining to avoid blood and tissue fluid collection in the immediate postoperative recovery period.

Abdominal wall closure: This is described in previous chapter on laparotomy.

References

Hiramatsu Y. (2019) Basic standard procedure of abdominal hysterectomy: Part 1. *Surg J (N Y)* **5**(Suppl 1): S2-S10. doi: 10.1055/s-0039-1678575.

Konishi I. (2018) Basic principle and step-by-step procedure of abdominal hysterectomy: Part 2. *Surg J (N Y)* **5**(Suppl 1): S11–S21. doi: 10.1055/s-0038-1676467.

Maresh MJ, Metcalfe MA, McPherson K, *et al.* (2002) The VALUE national hysterectomy study: Description of the patients and their surgery. *BJOG* **109**(3): 302–312. doi: 10.1111/j.1471-0528.2002.01282.x.

5

Vaginal Hysterectomy

Introduction

In vaginal hysterectomy, a surgery with no scars, the uterus is removed completely through a transvaginal surgical approach. It is a well-established procedure that is suitable for most cases of hysterectomy for benign pathology.

I had once received feedback from an overseas patient on whom I had 6 weeks previously performed a vaginal hysterectomy for heavy menstruation associated with uterine fibroids. She was extremely pleased with the totally unexpected ease of her surgical recovery. She had no postoperative pain that required any analgesia and was able to perform her daily physical activities immediately upon reaching home from the hospital. She told me that her official medical leave of 4 weeks for hysterectomy was one of the longest vacations that she had ever had during her working life, and further commented that her colleague's reaction to her remarkable recovery and absence of any surgical scars on her body did cast a doubt on her mind as to whether a hysterectomy had even been done. Of course, it was not difficult for me to assure her of the surgery with a surgicopathology report, complete with a full anatomical description of the hysterectomy specimen of the uterus.

In this chapter, the rationale and measures to overcome challenges of vaginal hysterectomy are presented. The surgical steps of a typical vaginal hysterectomy are described to illustrate the anatomical basis of the procedure. Variations of hysterectomy are described for salpingectomy, bilateral salpingo-oophorectomy, and laparoscopy-assisted vaginal hysterectomy.

The Benefits of Vaginal Hysterectomy Compared to Abdominal Hysterectomy

Vaginal hysterectomy is the least invasive form of hysterectomy as the route of surgery is a natural passage, without requiring even a single abdominal skin incision. Comparing vaginal hysterectomy to abdominal hysterectomy, a Cochrane review (2015) of nine randomized controlled trials involving 762 women reported a significantly shorter duration required to return to normal physical activities in favor of vaginal hysterectomy (mean difference was −9.5 days, 95% confidence interval of −12.6 to −6.4 days). There was no difference in this respect between vaginal hysterectomy and laparoscopic hysterectomy, but vaginal hysterectomy is associated with a significantly lower incidence of unintentional conversion to laparotomy.

Current evidence indicates that vaginal hysterectomy should be considered first before embarking on other types of hysterectomy.

Measures for Wider Adoption of Vaginal Hysterectomy

Against evidence-based medical practice, in reality, the frequency of vaginal hysterectomy today is less than 25% of all hysterectomy for benign pathology and the indication is nearly always for cases of uterovaginal prolapse. Several measures are necessary to correct the undeserved treatment the procedure has received thus far.

Gynecologist's Attitude

The nature of the surgery through a small vaginal canal limits visualization of the procedure for assistants and observers of vaginal hysterectomy. The unfamiliarity and negative impression of vaginal hysterectomy as a daunting procedure need to be expelled.

Gynecologist's Training

Comprehensive training in vaginal hysterectomy by experienced vaginal surgeons and clinical mentors is mandatory for acquisition of surgical techniques for vaginal hysterectomy. It also provides for resolving technical challenges during operations.

Public Awareness

Many women are unaware that hysterectomy can be done transvaginally as demonstrated by my patient and her colleagues in the narration earlier, leading many to accept other types of hysterectomy instead.

Indications of Vaginal Hysterectomy

Vaginal hysterectomy has had a long history since the era soon after the birth of Christ. At the time, it was performed to rectify an inverted uterus, which was a fatal obstetric complication. Although surgical risk then was as bad as the pathology with few survivors, it remained the better of the two evils. Today, indications for vaginal hysterectomy are based on pathological conditions that warrant removal of the uterus as detailed in Chapter 1. The practical question a gynecologist should really be asking is why a transvaginal hysterectomy should *not* be done.

Contraindication of Vaginal Hysterectomy

The selection of a vaginal route instead of laparotomy or laparoscopy is a consideration of technical feasibility. That is to say, gynecologists should be cognizant of the contraindications of vaginal hysterectomy. Vaginal hysterectomy is most frequently performed in the presence of uterovaginal prolapse, which is an extended rationale for the historic indication of the procedure for an inverted uterus. Today, the absence of uterine prolapse is not a contraindication for vaginal hysterectomy. Many factors or conditions are unfavorable but are not constitute absolute contraindications for vaginal hysterectomy. These are situations that increase the technical demands on the surgeon and the frequency of intraoperative alteration or conversion to laparoscopic assistance or laparotomy.

1. Inaccessibility of the uterus transvaginally
   — Uncorrectable vaginal stenosis from conditions such as previous vaginal surgery or severe postradiation fibrosis.
   — Vaginal or presacral tumors.
   — Orthopedic conditions that bar the patient from being placed in a lithotomy position with hip abduction.
2. Hysterectomy is part of other intra-abdominal procedures
   — Surgery for large ovarian cysts or tumors.
   — Hysterectomy in association with pelvic and/or para-aortic lymphadenectomy, typically for cancer of the cervix, endometrium, Fallopian tubes, ovary and omentum or peritoneum.

     — Surgery of the gastrointestinal tract, such as anterior resection of the colon, or appendicectomy.

     — Cesarean hysterectomy.

3. Unfavorable uterine conditions

     — Large uterine volume beyond the dimension of a 15-week gestation.

     — Previous myomectomy with suspected pelvic adhesions and dense fibrosis.

     — Morcellation or bisection of the uterus is contraindicated, such as endometrial carcinoma.

4. Unfavorable pelvic conditions

     — Known or suspected severe adhesions in the pelvis.

     — Severe pelvic endometriosis.

5. Unfavorable constitutional factors of the patient

     — Narrow subpubic arch (<90 degrees).

6. Patient's choice

     — Patient has a preference for other modes of hysterectomy.

Technique of Vaginal Hysterectomy

The surgical steps of a typical vaginal hysterectomy are described to illustrate the principles of the procedure. The detailed procedure is based on measures to optimize access to the uterus, application of precise anatomical knowledge, and principles of surgery aimed at achieving the lowest incidence of immediate and long-term complications.

Intraoperative Preparation

Anesthesia

Anesthesia with good relaxation of the vaginal and pelvic floor musculatures are essential for successful vaginal hysterectomy. Apart from general anesthesia, regional epidural or spinal anesthesia is appropriate as the innervation of the pelvic viscera and vagina-vulva-perineum derives from the low thoracolumbosacral nerve roots.

Instruments

Instruments for vaginal hysterectomy are evolving and many innovations, including new energy-based tissue sealing-and-cutting devices, endoloop sutures, surgical stapler devices, and laparoscopy-derived instruments, are helpful in various situations and to different surgeons. The key instruments adequate for the great majority of vaginal hysterectomies in my own set include:

(i) Vaginal wall retractors
  o Single-ended Sim speculum
  o Landon retractors
(ii) Curved Masterson artery forceps
(iii) Long dissecting forceps
  o Toothed forceps
  o Non-toothed forceps
(iv) Adhesive plastic vaginal drapes

Lithotomy position

The most optimal transvaginal access to the uterus is to put the patient in a dorsolithotomy position with a slight Trendelenburg tilt. The hips are partially abducted and the buttocks hang just over the edge of the operating table.

Vulvovaginal antisepsis

The skin preparation with povidone paint should cover the area extending from the lower abdomen to halfway down the thighs and the entire anogenital region. The vagina must also be thoroughly douched with the antiseptic.

After donning the legs and lower part of the body with sterile surgical drapes, the vulva and perineum are dabbed dry and sealed with an adhesive sterile plastic drape to separate the vagina from the anus.

Urinary drainage

The urinary bladder is emptied with an in-and-out catheter or a Foley's catheter, which can be retained for postoperative continuous drainage.

Steps of Vaginal Hysterectomy

Exposure of the Cervix

The vulva can be retracted laterally with a self-retaining retractor or maintained in lateral position with a surgical stitch on each side. A single-ended broad Sim's speculum or

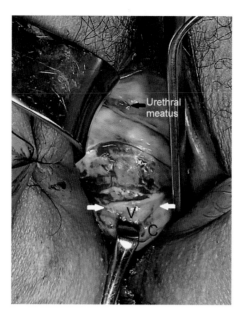

Figure 5.1 ■ A surgical photograph showing an incision made above the vaginocervical junction (marked by the two horizontal solid white arrows). "C" marks the smooth squamous mucosa of the ectocervix and "V" marks the anterior vaginal mucosa. The rugae is inconspicuous because of the postmenopausal status of the woman.

weighed Auvard speculum is used to expose the cervix. The cervix is firmly grasped with double-teethed vulsellum forceps at the 6 o'clock and 12 o'clock positions. The concave pelvic curvature of the vulsellum forceps faces ventrally to follow the natural axis of the uterovaginal canal.

The vaginocervix junction is a helpful surgical landmark for vaginal hysterectomy. It is the junction where the vagina mucosa with transverse rugae meets the smooth mucosa of the cervix (Figure 5.1). This surgical landmark is more prominent in the anterior vagina fornix. In the posterior fornix, the junction can be assumed to be at the level of a semicircular line connecting the right and left ends of the anterior border. The vaginocervical junction may be inconspicuous in postmenopausal women because of the loss of the vaginal rugae from estrogen withdrawal induced atrophy. Preoperative vaginal estrogen therapy improves its identification.

Preparation for Vaginal Incision

A gentle traction is applied to the vulsellum forceps to drag down the cervix and straighten the cervicouterine axis. Vaginal mucosa at the fornix distal to the vaginocervical junction is raised by submucosal infiltration of normal saline solution with or without diluted adrenalin (1:200,000) circumferentially around the cervix.

Posterior Vaginal Incision and Entering the Pouch of Douglas

The cervix is dragged anteriorly and the posterior vaginal wall retracted dorsally with a Sim's speculum to expose the posterior vaginal fornix under mild tension.

A V-shaped vaginal incision is made with a sharp scalpel. The two incision lines forming the "V" shape commence from the right and left lateral vaginocervical junction and converge to a point at the midline of the posterior vagina fornix, 1 to 2 cm distal to the posterior vaginocervical junction (Figure 5.2). Attention is needed to ensure that the incisions are perpendicular to the mucosa and complete in full thickness of the vaginal wall. The vagina mucosa is lifted up at the apex of the "V" with a pair of toothed dissecting forceps and reflected toward the vaginocervical junction. The raised flap of the vagina can be excised or included in the hold of the vulsellum forceps on the posterior cervix to ensure clear visualization of the surgical field.

The peritoneum in the pouch of Douglas can be seen to reflect on to the posterior cervix (Figure 5.3). It is grasped with toothed dissecting forceps and incised with sharp scissors. Scanty peritoneal fluid escapes vaginally. The peritoneal incision is enlarged by lateral stretching using index fingers and the peritoneal cavity is examined for the presence of adhesions and pathology.

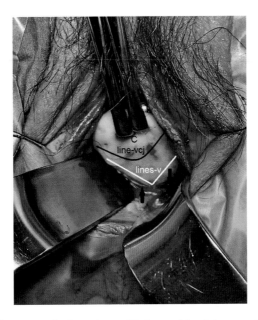

Figure 5.2 ■ A surgical photograph showing a V-shaped incision made on the posterior vaginal fornix. "C" indicates the posterior lip of the cervix; "line-vcj" indicates the position of the posterior vaginocervical junction; "lines-v" indicates the position of the V-shaped incision. The two solid black arrows indicate the two incisions of the V-shaped incision.

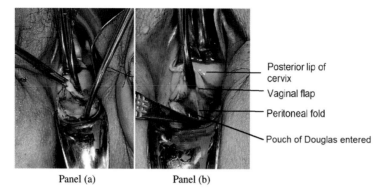

Panel (a)   Panel (b)

Figure 5.3 ■ Surgical photographs showing dissection (Panel (a)), grasping of the peritoneum of the pouch of Douglas, and incision into the pouch of Douglas (Panel (b)).

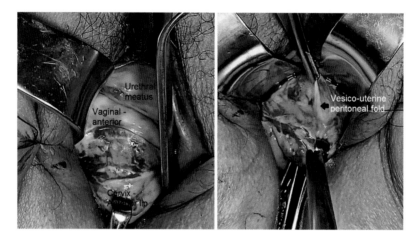

Figure 5.4 ■ A surgical photograph showing the peritoneum of the vesicouterine pouch lifted up in a forceps.

Anterior Circumcervical Incision and Opening of the Vesicocervical Space

An anterior circumcervical incision over the anterior vaginocervical junction is performed with a sharp scalpel, joining the two lines of the "V" incision laterally. With the cervix put under tension with mild downward and dorsal retraction, the vaginal wall is dissected away from the cervix, initially with scissors with the tips perpendicularly pressing onto the cervix in a "push away" action, followed by blunt dissection. The vesicocervical space is thus opened and the blunt dissection continues until the reflection of the vesicouterine peritoneum is encountered (Figure 5.4).

In the presence of dense adhesions and anatomical distortions from previous cesarean sections, vaginal hysterectomy in this part of the surgery carries an advantage over transabdominal hysterectomy. By commencing the dissection from a part not previously operated on, the transvaginal approach is always easier than having to start the dissection through dense adhesions in the abdominal approach.

Entering the Vesicouterine Pouch

The vesicocervical space is retracted ventrally with a right-angled Landon retractor to expose the line of peritoneal reflection between the urinary bladder and uterus. The loose part of the peritoneum between the peritoneal reflection line and bladder is picked up with a pair of toothed dissection forceps and incised with a pair of scissors (Figure 5.4). The glistening mucosal surface of the anterior wall of the uterus comes into view. The peritoneal incision is extended by stretching it laterally with index fingers.

In some cases with previous surgery such as a cesarean section, the indistinct border of the urinary bladder can be identified with a curved Hegar dilator. A size-5 Hegar dilator is introduced into the bladder through the urethra. With the concave side facing the anterior uterine wall and the tip gently pressed against the uterus, the dilator is moved toward the surgeon to indicate the border of the bladder.

Exposure of the Uterosacral and Cardinal Ligaments

The peritoneal cavity is kept open with a Landon retractor anteriorly and Sim's retractor posteriorly. The lateral vaginal wall is retracted away with a separate Landon retractor while the cervix is deviated toward the contralateral position. The incision edge of the vagina is pushed laterally to expose the cervical ends of the uterosacral and cardinal ligaments.

Uterosacral-cardinal Pedicle

The pedicles on the right- and left-hand sides are managed in the same manner. The entire thickness of the cervical portion of the uterosacral and cardinal ligaments are clamped with a pair of curved Masterson forceps (Figure 5.5). The tip of the clamping forceps is pressed onto the border of the cervix immediately inferior to the uterine artery. The pedicle is divided medially until the tip of the clamp is free from the cervix. The pedicle is ligated with a transfixing Vicryl-O suture and the cut end of the suture is anchored with a pair of mosquito forceps to the surgical drape at the side of the buttock.

Uterine Vessel Pedicles

Once the uterosacral and cardinal pedicles are divided, the uterus can be pulled further down into the vagina with little traction. The uterine vessels at the uterine border become

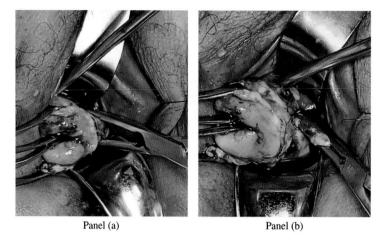

Panel (a)   Panel (b)

Figure 5.5 ■ Surgical photographs showing the placing of Masterson forceps on the uterosacral ligament (Panel (a)) and division of the pedicle (Panel (b))

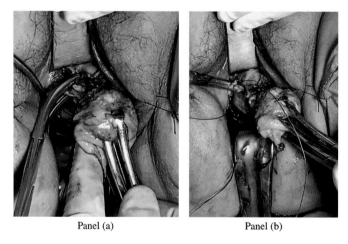

Panel (a)   Panel (b)

Figure 5.6 ■ Surgical photographs showing the placement of the Masterson clamps on the uterine vessels (Panel (a)) and division of the vessels (Panel (b)).

evident and are clamped with curved Masterson forceps. The tips of the Masterson forceps grasp the peritoneum in the vesicouterine space and the pouch of Douglas (Figure 5.6). The clamp should not include any part of the uterosacral-cardinal pedicle. The pedicle is divided with a sharp scalpel medially. The cervix and uterus are pushed up toward the pelvis to relieve obstructive occupation of the vagina by the uterus. This will improve access to the pedicle to facilitate its ligation. A transfixing suture with Vicryl-O is used to secure the pedicle. The knot is left free without traction.

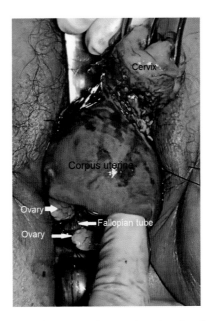

Figure 5.7 ■ A surgical photograph showing the uterine fundus being delivered out of the pelvis in a retroversion maneuver.

The Upper Uterine Pedicles

The uterus is pulled down and the broad ligament is trimmed at the lateral order of the uterus. With the uterus under downward traction, the ovarian ligament and round ligament are palpated to ensure freedom from bowel adhesions. The ovarian ligament, Fallopian tube, and round ligament are taken in a single pedicle using a pair of curved Masterson forceps and transected close to the border of the uterus (Figure 5.7). One of the vulsellum forceps on the cervix is freed to grasp the fundus of the uterus. Lateral traction of the uterus will display the contralateral round ligament, Fallopian tube, and ovarian ligament for clamping as described. Once these upper pedicles are transected, the uterus is free to be removed. The pedicle is ligated with a transfixing Vicryl-O suture. The cut ends of the suture are anchored with mosquito forceps to the surgical drape on the anterior aspect of the upper thigh.

Closure of Peritoneal Cavity

The pelvic cavity is explored and ovaries examined for any pathology. The purse-string suture with Vicryl-O suture is placed at the edge of the peritoneal incision. The suture is gently tightened while keeping a close watch to make sure that the Fallopian tubes do not prolapse out of the loop of the suture and enter the vagina. The completely tightened purse-string closes the peritoneal cavity with all the pedicles located in the extraperitoneal position.

The pedicle stumps and cut edges of all tissues are inspected meticulously for any bleeding. This is critical to ensure complete hemostasis.

Closure of Vaginal Vault

This process involves closure of the vaginal incision and attachment of the uterosacral-cardinal ligament pedicles to the vault. The pedicle attachment provides additional suspensory support to the upper vagina. This stepwise process proceeds as follows:

Preparation of pedicle attachment

The sutures holding the right and left uterosacral-cardinal pedicles are threaded through the full thickness of the vaginal wall at their respective lateral points of the vaginocervical junction. The free ends of the sutures are held with mosquito forceps.

Vaginal incision closure

The vaginal incision is closed in full thickness with a continuous locking Vicryl-O suture, starting from the apex of the "V" incision.

Suspension of the uterosacral-cardinal pedicles

The free ends of the right and left uterosacral-cardinal pedicle sutures held in the mosquito forceps are tied with a square knot across the midline of the vaginal vault.

Vaginal Tamponade

Routine application of a rolled surgical gauge pack or large vaginal tampon soaked in normal saline to provide vaginal tamponade for hemostasis is unnecessary.

Variations in Vaginal Hysterectomy

Vaginal Hysterectomy with Salpingectomy

Transvaginal access to salpingectomy is limited by the volume of the uterus. Intraoperative reduction of the uterine volume by myomectomy will facilitate the procedures. Two approaches are describe here.

Posterior delivery of the uterus for salpingectomy

After securing the uterine pedicles and division of the broad ligament to the insertion of ovarian ligaments bilaterally, the fundus of the uterus is pushed into the posterior vaginal fornix with the index finger in the vesicouterine pouch. The fundus is grasped with a pair of toothed tenaculum forceps. A downward and dorsal traction on the fundus, if necessary, with the cervix pushed into the vesicouterine pouch will expose the ovarian ligaments and the Fallopian tubes. These organs are inspected for any pathology.

The vaginal wall is retracted laterally with a pair of Landon forceps, the ovary is grasped with ovum forceps, and the ampulla of the Fallopian tube is picked up with dissecting forceps to put the mesosalpinx under mild tension. The mesosalpinx is divided close to the Fallopian tube toward the uterine insertion of the tube. The blood vessels encountered in the mesosalpinx are either tied off with sutures or sealed with electrodiathermy.

The ovarian ligament is clamped near the uterine border and ligated. The utero-ovarian blood vessels and round ligament can be clamped together in a single pedicle with a pair of curved Masterson forceps and transfixed with Vicryl-O suture.

In menopausal women with thin pedicles, the ovarian ligament, round ligament, and utero-ovarian blood vessels can be included in a single pedicle.

Salpingectomy after complete removal of the uterus

If the uterus is particularly obstructive in the vagina or the posterior delivery of the fundus is challenged by thick adenomyosis, the uterus can be completely removed in the same manner as that for routine vaginal hysterectomy as described in the earlier sections.

Any bowel loops that prolapse into the pouch of Douglas is pushed into the abdominal cavity with a surgical gauge wrapped using ovum forceps.

Division of the mesosalpinx for salpingectomy is then performed from the uterine end toward the infundibulopelvic ligament until the Fallopian tube is freed from the ovary.

Vaginal Hysterectomy with Bilateral Salpingo-oophorectomy

The uterine fundus is delivered into the posterior vaginal fornix as described above. The ovary is grasped with ovum forceps and retracted toward the vagina to display a segment of the infundibulopelvic ligament. After ensuring the absence of bowel adhesions, the infundibulopelvic ligament is clamped with a pair of curved Masterson forceps and divided. The pedicle is ligated with Vicryl-O sutures twice. The broad ligament is divided toward the border of the uterus. The ovarian ligament, utero-ovarian blood vessels, and round ligament can be clamped in one pedicle with curved Masterson forceps.

If the uterus has been completely removed, the broad ligament is divided toward the ovary. The ovary is retracted with a pair of ovum forceps to expose the segment of infundibulopelvic ligament for clamping and division as described earlier for salpingo-oophorectomy.

Vaginal Hysterectomy for a Uterus of Large Volume

When the uterus is enlarged by fibroids and the superior pedicle is not accessible from the vagina, the uterus is bisected and myomectomy is carried out or the thick myometrium from adenomyosis can be reduced with a coring procedure after securing uterosacral and uterine pedicles bilaterally.

To bisect the uterus, the vulsellum forceps are moved from the anterior and posterior lip of the cervix to the 3 o'clock and 9 o'clock positions of the cervix. The posterior vaginal wall is retracted with a Sim's speculum and the urinary bladder is retracted ventrally with a Landon retractor. The cervix is placed under downward and lateral tension and a longitudinal incision is made over the anterior and posterior walls. The incision is extended toward the uterine fundus until the uterus is totally divided into two halves. In the process, myomectomy is done by enucleation.

The superior pedicles of hysterectomy are performed on each side of the divided uterus individually, including salpingectomy or salpingo-oophorectomy as intended.

Laparoscopy-assisted Vaginal Hysterectomy

Laparoscopy-assisted vaginal hysterectomy (LAVH) was first performed by Dr Kurt Semm of the University of Kiel, Germany, in the early 1980s. This procedure combines the advantages of laparoscopy and vaginal hysterectomy to avoid the disadvantages of a laparotomy, such as its immediate and delayed risk of intraoperative complications.

It applies the advantage of laparoscopy during intraoperative evaluations of pelvic pathologies, such as the existence and extent of pelvic adhesions and endometriosis which challenge the success of blind entry of the pelvis in vaginal hysterectomy. It also allows efficient management of the superior uterine pedicles, Fallopian tubes, and ovaries. Thus, it enables transvaginal hysterectomy to be performed in many cases that would otherwise require a laparotomy. However, compared to vaginal hysterectomy, LAVH incurs longer operating time and risk of surgical complications for the additional laparoscopy procedure. Laparoscopy also allows inspection and hemostasis to be secured from the pelvic view before concluding the surgery, which reduces the incidence of vaginal vault hematoma.

In LAVH, creation of CO_2 pneumoperitoneum, introduction of the laparoscope, and siting of secondary ports for instrument introduction and manipulation are described in the chapter on laparoscopic total hysterectomy. The surgical technique for dealing with the superior pedicles of hysterectomy and/or salpingectomy and bilateral salpingo-oophorectomy is also performed in the same manner as in total laparoscopic hysterectomy. The broad ligament is divided to the level of insertion of uterosacral ligaments. The vesicouterine fold is incised and the vesicocervical space is dissected.

The management of inferior pedicles for the rest of hysterectomy follows from vaginal hysterectomy as described above. The uterus is bisected, if necessary, and removed transvaginally. The pelvic peritoneum and vaginal vault closure also follow the description on vaginal hysterectomy in earlier sections.

References

Aarts JWM, Nieboer TE, Johnson N, *et al.* (2015) Surgical approach to hysterectomy for benign gynaecological disease. *Cochrane Database Syst Rev* **8**: CD003677. DOI: 10.1002/14651858. CD003677.pub5.

Byrnes JN, Trabuco EC. (2016) Evidence basis for hysterectomy. *Obstet Gynecol Clin North Am* **43**(3): 495–515. doi: 10.1016/j.ogc.2016.04.009. PMID: 27521881.

Garry R, Fountain J, Mason S, *et al.* (2004) The eVALuate study: Two parallel randomised trials, one comparing laparoscopic with abdominal hysterectomy, the other comparing laparoscopic with vaginal hysterectomy. *BMJ* **328**(7432): 129–133.

Lee SH, Oh SR, Cho YJ, *et al.* (2019) Comparison of vaginal hysterectomy and laparoscopic hysterectomy: A systematic review and meta-analysis. *BMC Women's Health* **19**: 83.

Madhvani K, Curnow T, Carpenter T. (2019) Route of hysterectomy: a retrospective, cohort study in English NHS Hospitals from 2011 to 2017. *BJOG* **126**: 795–802.

Nieboer TE, Johnson N, Lethaby A, *et al.* (2009) Surgical approach to hysterectomy for benign gynaecological disease. *Cochrane Database Syst Rev* **3**: CD003677. DOI: 10.1002/14651858. CD003677.pub4.

Occhino JA, Gebhart JB. (2010) Difficult vaginal hysterectomy. *Clin Obstet Gynecol* **53**(1): 40–50. doi: 10.1097/GRF.0b013e3181ce8945.

Oláh K. (2005) Vaginal hysterectomy in the absence of prolapse. The Obstetrician & Gynaecologist **7**: 233–240.

Sandberg EM, Twijnstra ARH, Driessen SRC, *et al.* (2017) Total laparoscopic hysterectomy versus vaginal hysterectomy: A systematic review and meta-analysis. *J Minim Invasive Gynecol* **24**(2): 206–217.e22. doi: 10.1016/j.jmig.2016.10.020. Epub 2016 Nov 17. PMID: 27867051.

Stark M, Gerli S, di Renzo GC. (2006) Physicians should familiarize themselves with simpler methods for vaginal hysterectomy: The ten step vaginal hysterectomy. Progress in Obstetrics and Gynaecology **17**: 358–368.

Thurston J, Murji A, Scattolon S, *et al.* (2019) No. 377-Hysterectomy for benign gynaecologic indications. *J Obstet Gynaecol Can* **41**(4): 543–557. doi: 10.1016/j.jogc.2018.12.006. PMID: 30879487.

6

Laparoscopy for Hysterectomy

Introduction

Laparoscopy is an alternative to laparotomy and vaginal surgical approach to abdominal surgery. Its development aligns well with the quest to find the least traumatic way to conduct abdominal surgeries. As the nature of laparoscopy entails a wider change of practice than a sear alternative abdominal incision, adequate treatment of the subject is necessary before laparoscopic hysterectomy can be further described.

This chapter begins with a brief history of the development of laparoscopy while highlighting the challenges encountered and how they were overcome. This chapter provides readers a sound understanding and appreciation of the uniqueness of laparoscopy in nature, as well as its technique and complications in term of ergonomics and applied anatomy and physiology. It aims to enhance young gynecologists' confidence in considering the choice of laparoscopic hysterectomy. Also, this chapter draws attention of surgeons to the potential occupational health hazards associated with laparoscopic surgery.

The Development of Laparoscopy

Laparoscopy is a century-old surgical procedure, having existed since it was introduced in a publication by the Swedish surgeon Dr Hans Christian Jacobaeus in 1910. The development of the procedure has met with more opposition than any other surgical innovation in recent medical history. The procedure, limited by the properties of rudimentary instruments, was mainly diagnostic in nature. In retrospect, it is easy to understand the reasons for opposition and poor reception of laparoscopy from mainstream surgeons. During the era of poor anesthesiology, surgery was a high-risk endeavor justifiable only by its therapeutic intention. The concept of invasive surgery for diagnostic purposes was poorly received. The development of laparoscopy was further stunted by lack of scientific research to establish a defined role and clinical safety for it.

Laparoscopy was performed sporadically by a handful of enthusiastic surgeons in the ensuing 50 years. It crept into gynecologic surgery with the availability of a better forward-view laparoscope, insufflation of the peritoneal cavity, and electrocoagulation. Dr Boesch, a Swiss gynecologist, reported the first therapeutic laparoscopy for female sexual sterilization by coagulation of the Fallopian tubes in 1936. In 1947, Dr Raoul Palmer from France introduced the Veress needle for pneumoperitoneum. The needle was invented by Dr János Veress in 1932 to induce pneumothorax to collapse the lungs during treatment of tuberculosis. Dr Palmer further expanded laparoscopy surgery to adhesiolysis, hemostasis by coagulation and puncturing of the ovarian cysts in the 1950s and 1960s, and ovum retrieval for in-vitro fertilization in 1971. He also described, in 1974, a safe laparoscopy insertion point 3 cm below the tip of the last rib in the upper-left quadrant of the abdomen, known as the Palmer's point. The leap of therapeutic laparoscopy since the 1960s has been accredited to Dr Kurt Semm, a German gynecologist. He developed laparoscopic surgical instruments, such as an automated pneumatic-CO_2 insufflator, Fallopian tube insufflation devices, and intra- and extra-corporeal knot tying techniques, and performed a variety of gynecological surgeries, including laparoscopy-assisted vaginal hysterectomy. He was one of the most prolific laparoscopic surgeons for 40 years, but he met with strong opposition and severe criticism during his earlier years, being viewed as an errant surgeon not fit for medical practice, which nearly terminated his professional career.

In early 1980s, Dr Camran Nehzat, a gynecologist from New York, improved the ergonomic property of laparoscopic surgery by coupling a camera attached to the eye piece of a laparoscope to a monitor. The subsequent development and wide availability of chip-based, high-quality video cameras brought laparoscopic surgery to new heights of interest in gynecology and other surgical disciplines. The first total hysterectomy performed completely through laparoscopy was reported in 1988 by Dr Harry Reich, an American gynecologist in Pennsylvania.

The Early Era of Laparoscopy in Clinical Practice

In the United Kingdom, laparoscopy was popularized in the 1970s by Dr Patrick Steptoe, a British obstetrician and gynecologist who, together with Professor Robert Edwards, pioneered in-vitro fertilization in Oldham General Hospital and Bourn Hall Clinic in Cambridgeshire, UK. He had learned laparoscopy from Dr Raoul Palmer in 1967.

Laparoscopy has since established itself in routine gynecology in the UK. Laparoscopy with Veress needle insufflation of CO_2 to create pneumoperitoneum was introduced to me on my first day of residency training in the early 1980s. It was routinely used for diagnosis of conditions causing relenting or recurrent pelvic pain and had largely replaced hysterosalpingograms for assessment of Fallopian tube patency. Its therapeutic role was largely for Fallopian tube occlusion for sexual sterilization and treatment of subfertility, including ova retrieval, gamete transfer, and intratubal insemination of sperm. By then, electrodiathermy cauterization of Fallopian tubes had become uncommon. Band-ligation (Falope ring) of the Fallopian tubes was also being rapidly replaced by self-locking clips (Filsie clips).

The Uniqueness of Laparoscopy

Instead of a large incision on the abdominal wall in laparotomy, small incisions or punctures are made at appropriate locations over the anterior abdominal wall to insert viewing telescopes and operating instruments into the peritoneal cavity and to remove resected tissues or organs. In this respect, laparoscopic surgery fulfills the concept of the basic principle of surgery — by introducing the least iatrogenic trauma to the anatomy and physiology to minimize factors that go against the natural law of healing. In addition, the accessibility of a thin telescope to different parts of the intra-abdominal and pelvic cavity and retroperitoneal spaces under a safe pressure-sustained pneumoperitoneum cavity provides the operation team an excellent view of the entire surgical field. The built-in brilliant light illumination and magnified view of the telescope system enable the surgical dissection, resection, and placement of suture ligatures and hemostasis to be carried out with great anatomical precision. Compared to laparotomy surgery, the apparent lesser invasiveness of laparoscopic surgery has resulted in the emergence of a whole new specialty known as minimally invasive surgery in recent years. The feasibility of laparoscopy has been proven for almost all known abdominal, pelvic, and cardiothoracic surgeries. The concept and practice of laparoscopic surgery have further extended to nearly all types of surgery outside body cavities.

Clinical experience over the last few decades has indeed proven that minimally invasive laparoscopic surgery expedites the healing process. Its advantage over open or laparotomy surgery is reflected in clinical benefits to patients, such as lesser severity and shorter duration of postoperative pain, earlier resumption to physical activities, lower incidence of complications related to prolonged physical inactivity, better healing and cosmetic appearance of surgical wounds, and shorter duration of hospital stay. These advantages also translate to financial benefits to patients and society at large.

The unique nature of laparoscopic surgery is seen in four broad aspects:

Surgical Skill Development and Adaptation

Therapeutic laparoscopic surgery largely adopts traditional open surgical procedures. Most of the steps of surgery, say in a total hysterectomy, are similar between the approaches for laparotomy and laparoscopy. However, the nature of laparoscopy requires unique modification of surgical techniques and acquisition of new surgical skill sets.

Psychovisual orientation

The view of the surgical field is transmitted via a monovision telescope through a video camera to a monitor. The two-dimensional image of the surgical field on the screen results in a rather virtual experience of the surgical maneuver compared to the conventional three-dimensional binocular vision of direct open surgery. There is a psychovisual learning process to facilitate adaptation to this new image experience.

Proprioception orientation

Proprioception learning is needed to correct surgeons' orientation of hand positioning and movements given that they are relying on images on a monitor screen some distance away from the actual surgical operative field, as well as having altered body and arm postures while handling laparoscopic surgical instruments. The learning process also involves adapting to the loss of direct tactile and force sensation when operating through laparoscopy.

Psychomotor dexterity

In addition to viewing surgical filed on a virtual projection and dealing with altered proprioception, laparoscopic surgeons' psychomotor dexterity is further aggravated by the demands of different hand, wrist, and finger maneuvers on handling laparoscopic instruments on one hand and the need to coordinate foot movements to control the pedal switches of energy delivery systems on the other hand. Not surprisingly, the most significant part of the learning curve for laparoscopic surgical tasks revolves around the acquisition of new motor dexterity.

Maintenance of Sustained Pneumoperitoneum

Together with appropriate positioning of the patient, sustained pneumoperitoneum keeps the peritoneal and pelvic cavity sufficiently distended and the bowel loops clear of the field of operation.

Safe procedures for the creation of pneumoperitoneum and maintenance of optimal intra-abdominal pneumatic pressure are a core skill of good laparoscopists.

Ergonomics of Laparoscopic Surgery

Laparoscopic surgical ergonomics play a critical role in the performance of surgeons, clinical outcomes and safety of surgery, and whether surgeons' health is compromised. The important contributing factors to ergonomic challenges specific to laparoscopic surgery include:

Environmental factors

The system set-up of the operating room for laparoscopic surgery involves stacks of electronic devices for video camera transmission, monitors for visual displays, intra-abdominal gas delivery and evacuation, and surgical energy delivering systems for tissue coagulation, sealing, and cutting. The physical arrangement of these systems in the operating room and the quality of performance of the systems directly influence the performance and safety of surgery. A well-designed, purpose-built operating room for laparoscopy is much desired but practically unavailable currently in most surgical facilities worldwide. Surgeons are left to adapt their existing operating environment as needed for laparoscopic surgery.

Patient factors

Laparoscopic procedures are performed through instrument access ports at fixed and limited locations. Patient factors like physical build, such as gross obesity or being underweight, as well as the type and dimension of pathology can significantly affect surgical performance by limiting the range of surgical maneuvers and increasing the potential risk of injury to viscera and neurovascular structures. Appropriate positioning of the patient and the operating table is critically important in mitigating the challenges that may arise from the patient's body and physical state.

Instrument factors

The speed with which conventional open surgery has transformed to laparoscopic surgery in the last few decades is a direct consequence of new developments in laparoscopic instruments. They include the adaptation of conventional surgical forceps and scissors to fit laparoscopic operating channels, as well as the development of novel energy-based surgical devices, mechanical tissue sealing clips, tissue removal devices, and efficient systems to maintain smoke-free pneumoperitoneum and clear vision of the surgical field. Innovative uterine manipulators that use a Koh ring pneumo-occluder to prevent loss of pneumoperitoneum on colpotomy, for example, enable total hysterectomy to be performed completely by laparoscopy.

In addition to understanding the functional properties and modes of action of these instruments, surgeons must choose instruments with good design and quality to achieve desired performance.

Surgeon factors

Surgical skill is a function of time exposure and practice. Most surgeons experience a short learning curve for laparoscopic surgery, but there are several surgeon-specific constraints and challenges. Most importantly, physical health and strength are needed for surgeons to cope with the physical fatigue induced by adopting an unnatural posture with elevated arm positions to accommodate the fixed locations of the operative instrument ports. The low ratio of the surgeon's bodily height and arm length to the patient's bodily thickness and width adds to the physical demands on the surgeon. Currently available laparoscopic instruments are limited in choice for dimensions and weight and may be suboptimal for the size of hands and fingers of some surgeons. The impact of these factors is exacerbated by the complexity and duration of surgery.

A surgeon's physical fatigue directly impacts the performance of surgery. Equally, suboptimal ergonometric factors increase the risk of health hazards, in particular musculoskeletal disorders, for laparoscopic surgeons.

Laparoscopic Surgical Complications

Surgical complications

In additional to the generic risk of surgical complications related to the anatomy and pathology of surgical conditions, laparoscopy also carries a rare but unique risk of complications from pneumoperitoneum creation and trocar introduction, in particular injuries to intra-abdominal viscera and major vascular structures in the anterior abdominal wall, pelvic side walls, and retroperitoneal spaces posteriorly.

Abnormal gas distribution

Insufflation of gas to create pneomoperitoneum may result in abnormal distribution of gas in subcutaneous tissue in the form of emphasema or more catastrophic gas embolism.

Cardiovascular and respiratory embarrassment

Raised intra-abdominal pressure caused by pneomoperitoneum induces changes in cardiac output which may compromise hemodynamic status in vulneerable patients.

Ventilatory emabarrassment may arise from splinting effects of raised intra-abdominal pressure on the diaphragm.

Body acid-base imbalance

Respiratory acidosis may result from excessive absorption of carbon dioxide gas in a prolonged surgery.

Well-leg compartment syndrome

Ischemic muscle injury with myolysis from compromised blood flow to the elevated lower limps may occur in laparoscopy surgery.

Surgical Pelvic Anatomy for Laparoscopy

Besides specific pathological conditions, anatomical structure determines the appropriate choice of locations for the creation of pneumoperitoneum and introduction of instruments.

Structural Composition and Thickness of the Abdominal Wall

The umbilicus, a scar resulting from the severance of the umbilical cord at birth, is the most important surgical landmark on the anterior abdominal wall in laparoscopy. The central part of the umbilicus, known as the umbilicus tip, is the direct remnant of the umbilicus cord. This is surrounded by the umbilical collar which is a fibrous tissue of the umbilical ring, an embryonic structure through which the embryonic mid-gut migrates. The fibrous tissue of the umbilical ring is continuous with the fibrous tissue of the rectal sheath. The immediate abdominal skin surrounding the umbilicus may form a fold known as the umbilical hood.

The subcutaneous compartment of the anterior abdominal wall are layers of adipose tissue separated by the superficial Camper's fascia and the deeper and more fibrous Scarpa's fascia. Scarpa's fascia fuses with the linea alba at the midline and the fascia lata below the inguinal ligament. The thickness of the subcutaneous adipose tissue layer is the thinnest at the umbilicus. This is the universally accepted site for the primary port of entry into the peritoneal cavity in laparoscopy.

Between individuals, the umbilicus assumes a variety of shapes on the surface of the abdominal skin, ranging from being flat, recessed, or protruded. In anatomy, the umbilicus is described as located on the midline of the central part of the anterior abdominal wall, where the skin is innervated by the 10th thoracic nerve and is directly opposite the vertebral level between L3 and L4. The bifurcation of the abdominal aorta is located immediately in front of the vertebral body at this level. Uncontrolled vertical movement of instruments at the umbilicus risks injury of the aorta.

Vascular Structures in the Anterior Abdominal Wall

The main vascular structure of the anterior abdominal wall is the epigastric vascular system comprising inferior and superior epigastric arteries and veins. The inferior epigastric artery is larger in caliber than the superior epigastric artery. This vascular system provides significant collateral blood circulation to the lower limbs in the presence of vascular occlusion in the proximal iliac arteries. Injuries to these vessels cause severe hemorrhage and hematoma formation in the rectus abdominis muscles.

The inferior epigastric artery arises as a branch of the external iliac artery at the level of the inguinal canal (Figure 6.1). Its anatomical origin is immediately medial to the deep inguinal ring, and it courses anteromedially along the lateral border of the rectus abdominis muscle. At the level of the arcuate line, located halfway between the umbilicus and symphysis pubis, it enters the rectus abdominis muscle and continues its course cranially within the muscle. At the level of the umbilicus, it anastomoses with the superior epigastric artery (Figure 6.2).

The superior epigastric artery is the terminal branch of the internal mammary artery. Its course below the level of the diaphragm lies between the transversalis fascia and the

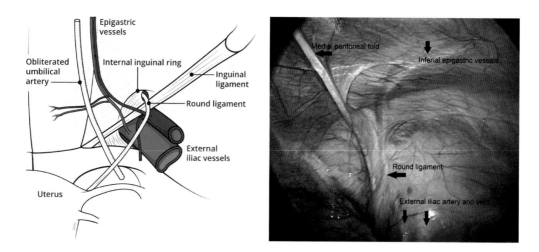

Figure 6.1 ■ The sketch (on the left) illustrates the origin of inferior epigastric vessels from the external iliac vessels and their anatomical relationship to the internal inguinal ring, round ligament, and obliterated umbilical artery. The anatomical relationship is further shown in the surgical photograph (on the right).

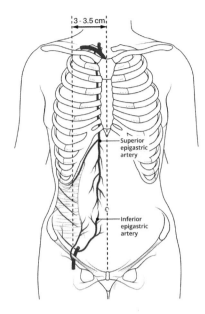

Figure 6.2 ■ An illustration of the territory of the inferior epigastric artery and its anastomosis with the superior epigastric artery at the level of the umbilicus.

rectus abdominis muscle. In the epigastric region, it penetrates the rectus abdominis muscle and ends with anastomosis with the inferior epigastric artery. The distribution of the main branches of epigastric arteries is confined to the central part of the abdomen within a 5 cm zone on either side of the midline.

Vascular Structures in the Lateral Pelvic Walls

The iliac blood vessels are the main vascular structures on the lateral wall of the pelvis. The abdominal aorta bifurcates at the level of the fourth lumbar vertebra into the right and left common iliac arteries. At the level of the sacroiliac joint approximately 4 cm lateral to the midline of the sacral promontory, the common iliac artery divides into the external and internal branches (Figure 6.3). The external iliac artery takes its course along the border of the pelvic portion of the psoas muscle and exits the pelvis through the femoral ring.

The internal iliac artery courses posterocaudally and divides into the anterior branch to supply the pelvic visceral structures and the posterior branch to supply the perineum. The anterior branch gives rise to the uterine artery and terminates as the umbilical artery. The umbilical artery is divided into the supravesical branch to supply the superior portion of the urinary bladder and the distal portion of the ureter, and the umbilical cord artery during fetal life. The umbilical cord artery thromboses after cutting of the cord at birth and becomes obliterated.

External iliac veins enter the pelvis through the femoral rings and are located medial to the corresponding external iliac arteries. In the remaining course in the cephalad

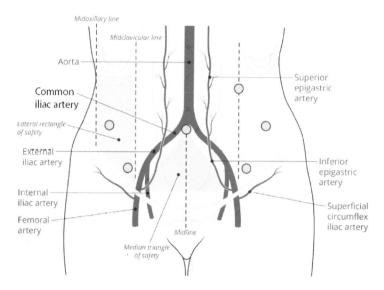

Figure 6.3 ■ An illustration of the relationship of the vascular supply to pelvic structures and the anterior abdominal wall.

direction, the right external iliac vein turns inferior, passes under the right external iliac artery, and lies lateral to it to become the common iliac vein at the pelvic brim. The left external iliac vein remains medioinferior to the left external iliac artery and turns medially at the pelvic brim. It then crosses the midline above the sacral promontory to join the right common iliac vein at the 5th vertebral level to form the inferior vena cava.

Vascular Structures Posterior to the Abdominal Peritoneum

The median (or middle) sacral artery branches off from the posterior aspect of the abdominal aorta immediately before it bifurcates into the common iliac arteries. It crosses anterior to the midline of the sacral promontory to enter the pelvis along the sacral curve to supply the sacrum and coccyx.

Abdominal Surface Anatomical Landmarks for Laparoscopic Hysterectomy Port Locations

The Umbilical Hood

This marks the inferior caudal border of the fibrous umbilical collar where the abdominal wall is thinnest. This is the preferred location to insert a Veress needle for the creation of pneumoperitoneum.

The Subumbilical Median "Triangle of Safety"

A triangular part of the central portion of the lower abdomen can be defined by two oblique lines joining the umbilicus to the midpoints of the inguinal ligaments (Figure 6.3). This triangular zone marks a region of the abdominal wall between the right and left inferior epigastric vessels on the anterior abdominal wall and right and left iliac vessels on the lateral pelvic walls. Deviation of the Veress needle and trocar beyond this triangular range during insertion may result in vascular injury.

The Right and Left Lateral "Zones of Safety"

These are two lateral portions of the anterior abdomen wall each flanked by the mid-clavicular and mid-axillary lines on the right and left side of the abdomen respectively (Figure 6.3). The mid-clavicular line is approximately 5 cm lateral to the alba linea at the epigastric region and 7 cm at the level of the umbilicus. Being lateral to the rectus abdominis muscles and epigastric vessels, these lateral zones of the abdomen are suitable as laparoscopic port locations to avoid vascular injury.

The Palmer's Point

In his original description, Palmer advocated insertion of Veress needle at a point 3 cm below the tip of the left 12th rib. This so-called Palmer's point falls within the upper end of the left lateral rectangular zone of safety for Veress needle insertion. The main structures in this part of the abdomen are gastrointestinal viscera (Figure 6.4).

Applied Physiology for Laparoscopy

Effects of Pressure of Pneumoperitoneum

The peritoneal cavity has a relatively low mean intra-abdominal pressure (IAP) of 5 to 7 mmHg. An elevated IAP of 12 to 20mm Hg is defined as intra-abdominal hypertension. Sustained pressure of more than 20 mmHg, defined as abdominal compartmental syndrome, is associated with serious organ dysfunction or failure.

During operative gynecologic laparoscopy, the automated pneumoperitoneum insufflator apparatus measures CO_2 flow pressure rather than the actual IAP. Clinical measurements taken 4 minutes after CO_2 insufflation at a flow pressure between 11 mmHg and 15 mmHg showed a marked increase in heart rate, systemic blood pressure,

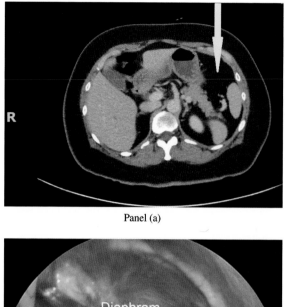

Panel (a)

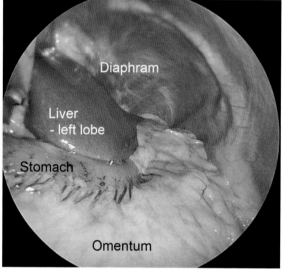

Panel (b)

Figure 6.4 ■ Panel (a) shows the abdominal viscera at Palmer's point on a CT scan. Panel (b) is a surgical photograph showing a laparoscopic view of the region of Palmer's point.

and central venous pressure among women undergoing a laparoscopic tubal sterilization procedure. There was also an increase in $PaCO_2$ and hydrogen ions. These changes are related to reduced compliance of the anterior abdominal wall, elevated level and reduced movement of the diaphragm, compression of the inferior vena cava, reduced blood circulatory return to the heart, and activated neurohormonal and renin-angiotensin responses. Compared to lower intra-abdominal pressure, a pressure above 15 mmHg is associated with more postoperative pain at 24 hours after surgery. The impact of these physiological changes can be expected to increase with the duration of sustained insufflation pressure and degree of Trendelenburg position.

The tamponade effect of pneumoperitoneum may mask venous injuries and insidious retroperitoneal venous bleeding. Any continuous bleeding after gaseous decompression may result in immediate or early postoperative hemodynamic decompensation and compromises.

The compliance of the anterior abdominal wall to reduce abdominal movement from the thrust pressure of a trocar insertion is achieved when the insufflation flow pressure is maintained at 25 mmHg. This has become the widely accepted level of pressure for the brief moment of trocar insertion. The insufflation flow pressure is then reduced to between 10 mmHg and 15 mmHg to maintain a clear operative field.

Effects of Types of Gas

The ideal gas for laparoscopic surgery should be colorless to provide a clear and untinted visual field, nonflammable and nonexplosive with surgical applications of electrodiathermy or other energy devices, nontoxic to patients, easily excreted, and easily available at low cost.

Carbon dioxide

CO_2 is the standard gas for laparoscopy since the 1920s. It is colorless and chemically stable, with a high diffusion capacity and solubility that allow it to be rapidly absorbed and excreted via ventilation. There is, however, a potential risk of hypercarbia and acidosis with resultant tachycardia, cardiac arrhythmias, and pulmonary edema. CO_2 peritoneal irritation is believed to contribute to postoperative pain.

Inert gases

Helium and argon are colorless and chemically inert gases. Clinical data comparing these inert gases to CO_2 is scarce and insufficient to demonstrate any differences in cardiopulmonary effects. Available data shows a tendency for lower pain scores among users of helium than those who use CO_2 gas pneumoperitoneum. Helium and argon are less soluble than CO_2 and have been reported to be associated with a higher incidence of subcutaneous emphysema. It is, theoretically, more likely to cause gas embolism than CO_2.

Nitrous oxide

At room temperature, nitrous oxide (N_2O) is a colorless gas. It is tasteless but has a mild sweet odor. After absorption, it is carried in the form of a solution in the blood. It has a mild analgesic effect and is widely known as a laughing gas. It is nonflammable but facilitates the combustion of oxygen. Available but limited comparative clinical data shows little difference in cardiopulmonary effects between N_2O and CO_2 pneumoperitoneum. A tendency toward lower pain scores has been reported among patients who had N_2O pneumoperitoneum compared to patients who had CO_2 pneumoperitoneum. Rare case reports of explosion during electrocautery surgery raise controversy over its safety in routine laparoscopic surgery.

Room air

There is a recent research interest on the potential use of room air, which is abundantly available at low cost, for pneumoperitoneum during laparoscopic surgery. The available clinical data comparing room air to CO_2 is scarce and inconclusive.

Contraindications for Laparoscopy

Some conditions impose additional technical, time, and resource demands for laparoscopy. Other conditions may expose the patient to additional risks of surgical complications when performed laparoscopically compared to open surgery. They constitute what are commonly known as contraindications for laparoscopy, most of which are relative rather than absolute contraindications. These factors come from pathologic, patient, and coexisting medical conditions.

Pathologic Conditions

Successful laparoscopy surgery has been used to treat almost all types of benign and malignant gynecological pathologies confined to the pelvis. Currently, the accepted contraindications for laparoscopic surgery include:

Radical hysterectomy for invasive cervical carcinoma

Clinical evidence indicates an increased hazard ratio for disease relapses and mortality among patients treated with laparoscopic radical hysterectomy compared to equivalent conventional laparotomy surgery.

Ovarian cystectomy for cystic tumors with suspected malignancy

Rupture of malignant cystic tumors, by disseminating tumor cells in the cyst content, upstages the ovarian cancer and compromises the potential curability of the tumor.

Pelvic Anatomical Conditions

Physical constrain that may prevent safe entry into or create inadequate working space in the abdomen. These constrains may arise from:

— Severe pelvic adehsions
— Obstructive leiomyomata
— Anatomical limitation
— History of repeat caesarean sections, multiple laparotomies, or midline incisions

Patient-specific Comorbidities

Some co-morbidities on the patient may not be suitable for laparosccopic surgery. These include:

— Cardiovascular diseases
— Raised intra-cranial pressure
— End-stage renal failure
— Uncorrected hypovolemia

Risk Factors Prompting Conversion to Laparotomy

Laparoscopic surgery is sometimes challenged by conditions that render it less safe than an open surgery. Under these circumstances, the laparoscopic approach is abandoned and the surgery proceeds with an open laparotomy as the alternative. Some predictors for the potential conversion of laparoscopy to open laparotomy include:

— elevated BMI rendering the creation of pneumoperitoneum difficult with either a Veress needle or open technique for trocar entry,
— increased uterine width greater than 10 cm,
— lateral or lower uterine segment fibroids that are over 5 cm,
— previous adhesion-forming abdominopelvic surgery.

Patients should be adequately counselled and they should provide consent for conversion of laparoscopy to laparotomy before the final decision to conduct laparoscopic hysterectomy is made.

Risk of Postsurgery Peritoneal Adhesions

Peritoneal adhesions occur commonly after intra-abdominal and pelvic surgeries. A small but significant group of these patients suffers serious morbidity and requires repeat surgeries, mainly for bowel obstructions. The etiology and mechanism of adhesion formation is complex and not yet fully understood. It is a common belief among surgeons that laparoscopy may be associated with less peritoneal adhesions and less frequent adhesion-related morbidities. A large Scottish epidemiology study provided evidence that the incidence of hospital readmission for adhesion-related reasons was similar between gynecologic laparoscopy and laparotomy.

References

Desimone CP, Ueland FR. (2008) Gynecologic laparoscopy. *Surg Clin North Am* **88**(2): 319–341, vi. doi: 10.1016/j.suc.2007.12.008.

Hayden P, Cowman S. (2011) Anaesthesia for laparoscopic surgery. *CEACCP* **11**: 177–180.

Jiménez AM, Colomer AT. (2008) An update of anatomical references in total laparoscopic radical hysterectomy: from surgical anatomy to anatomical surgery. *J Minim Invasive Gynecol* **15**(1): 4–10. doi: 10.1016/j.jmig.2007.07.009.

Kadar N. (1996) Surgical anatomy and dissection techniques for laparoscopic surgery. *Curr Opin Obstet Gynecol* **8**(4): 266–277.

Kyle EB, Maheux-Lacroix S, Boutin A, *et al.* (2015) Complications of low compared to standard pneumoperitoneum pressures in laparoscopic surgery for benign gynecologic pathology: a systematic review protocol. *Syst Rev* **4**: 96.

Llarena NC, Shah AB, Milad MP. (2015) Bowel injury in gynecologic laparoscopy: a systematic review. *Obstet Gynecol* **125**: 1407–1417.

Lower AM, Hawthorn RJ, Clark D, *et al.* (2004) Adhesion-related readmissions following gynaecological laparoscopy or laparotomy in Scotland: an epidemiological study of 24,046 patients. *Hum Reprod* **19**(8): 1877–1885. doi: 10.1093/humrep/deh321. Epub 2004 Jun 3. PMID: 15178659.

Marshall RL, Jebson PJR, Davie IT, *et al.* (1972) Circulatory effects of carbon dioxide insufflation of the peritoneal cavity and laparoscopy. *Brit J Anaesth* **44**: 680.

Ott DE. (2008) Laparoscopy and adhesion formation, adhesions and laparoscopy. *Semin Reprod Med* **26**(4): 322–330. doi: 10.1055/s-0028-1082390. PMID: 18756409.

Ott DE. (2019) Abdominal compliance and laparoscopy: a review. *JSLS* **23**: e2018.00080

Sánchez-Margallo FM, Sánchez-Margallo JA. (2017) Ergonomics in laparoscopic surgery. Laparoscopic Surgery Edit. Malik A. 2017; pp. 1787

Yu T, Cheng Y, Wang X, *et al.* (2017) Gases for establishing pneumoperitoneum during laparoscopic abdominal surgery. *Cochrane Database Syst Rev* **6**: CD009569. DOI: 10.1002/14651858.CD009569.pub3.

7

Laparoscopic Hysterectomy Procedure

Introduction

Laparoscopic hysterectomy refers to hysterectomy involving the use of a laparoscope. It was first introduced by Dr Kurt Semm to overcome technical challenges encountered during vaginal hysterectomy that would otherwise warrant an abdominal hysterectomy. Some examples of these challenges include history of previous pelvic surgeries, adhesions, severe endometriosis, or nulliparous women with limited vaginal access for hysterectomy. In 1988, Dr Harry Reich from Pennsylvania introduced the concept and conducted the first recorded case of total laparoscopic hysterectomy (TLH) in place of abdominal hysterectomy. Indeed, in the UK, the frequency of laparoscopic hysterectomy has surpassed all other single modes of hysterectomy to reach a proportion of 47% in 2017. This rise was most marked for the disease category of endometrial carcinoma compared to other benign conditions of the uterus.

The main content of this chapter includes: (1) definitions of different types of laparoscopic hysterectomy; (2) evidence-based information on the merits and shortcomings of laparoscopic hysterectomy; (3) technical details on how to safely create an optimal pneumoperitoneum; and (4) a description of the surgical procedure for laparoscopic hysterectomy. The objective information presented here allows for informed discussions between gynecologists and women considering hysterectomy, while the technical details of the surgical procedure help to illustrate the maneuvers involved in laparoscopic hysterectomy.

Classification of Laparoscopic Hysterectomy

Due to the extent of surgical procedures accomplished laparoscopically, the literature on laparoscopic hysterectomy contains a wide variety of terminology. In essence, there are four broad types of laparoscopic hysterectomy in current gynecologic practice:

Laparoscopy-assisted Vaginal Hysterectomy

In laparoscopy-assisted vaginal hysterectomy (LAVH), laparoscopic surgical procedures operate on the upper pedicles during hysterectomy and include:

— Clearing the surgical field in the pelvis — lysis of fibrotic or other visceral adhesions and excision of endometriosis, if any;
— Ligation and severance of either the infundibulopelvic ligaments or ovarian ligaments;
— Dissection of Fallopian tubes from the ovaries, if necessary; and
— Ligation and severance of round ligaments.
— The remaining surgical steps of hysterectomy are performed through a transvaginal route as in vaginal hysterectomy.

Laparoscopic Hysterectomy

In laparoscopic hysterectomy, laparoscopic procedures extend from those in LAVH to include:

— Laparoscopic cutting and ligation of uterine vessels;
— Performing the remaining surgical steps of hysterectomy through the vaginal route.

Total Laparoscopic Hysterectomy

— Total laparoscopic hysterectomy involves all the surgical steps of hysterectomy as described above plus performing the closure of the vaginal vault laparoscopically.

Laparoscopic Supracervical Hysterectomy

— The entire surgical procedure of hysterectomy up to the level of the main branch of the uterine arteries is performed laparoscopically. The cervix is conserved and the uterus is removed by morcellation.

Comparison Between Laparoscopic Hysterectomy, Vaginal Hysterectomy, and Abdominal Hysterectomy

There is ongoing discussion among gynecologic surgeons on the merits and demerits of abdominal, vaginal, and laparoscopic hysterectomy, and each procedure is not short of advocates. Existing evidence-based information from clinical trials provides a good basis for understanding the characteristics of each type of hysterectomy objectively.

Randomized controlled trials between 1996 and 2000 in the UK compared laparoscopic hysterectomy (predominantly the LAVH type) to abdominal hysterectomy for benign uterine diseases in the absence of pelvic organ prolapse of grade 3 or more severe and where the uterine size did not exceed 12-week gestations. Ray Garry and co-authors reported that laparoscopic hysterectomy had an advantage over abdominal hysterectomy with a shorter mean duration of hospital stay (3 days versus 4 days) and better quality of life at 6 weeks postsurgery. The advantage of laparoscopic hysterectomy disappeared only after 12 months postsurgery. On the other hand, laparoscopic hysterectomy required a longer operating time (84 minutes versus 50 minutes) and carried a 3.9% incidence of unintended laparotomy. Furthermore, compared to abdominal hysterectomy, laparoscopic hysterectomy carried a higher chance of encountering at least one major complication (11.1% versus 6.2%), specifically major hemorrhage (4.6% versus 2.4%), intra-abdominal visceral injuries (3.2% versus 2%), and major anesthetic complications (0.9% versus none).

The same researchers conducted a randomized controlled trial on laparoscopic hysterectomy and vaginal hysterectomy during the same study period with similar inclusion criteria. They found that there was no discernible difference between the two modes of hysterectomy in median duration of hospital stay (3 days), quality of life at 6 weeks or at 12 months postsurgery, incidence of at least one major complication (9.8% versus 9.5%), and visceral injuries (1.2%). Laparoscopic hysterectomy , however, took a longer operation time (72 minutes versus 39 minutes) while vaginal hysterectomy had a higher rate of unintended laparotomy (4.2% versus 2.7%).

A meta-analysis of 18 randomized controlled trials published between 2000 and 2018 reported that there was no difference between overall complication rate, rate of conversion to laparotomy, length of hospital stay, and recuperation time between vaginal hysterectomy and LAVH, between vaginal hysterectomy and TLH, and between vaginal hysterectomy and laparoscopic hysterectomy (unspecified type). Vaginal hysterectomy, however, consistently showed a superiority to all types of laparoscopic hysterectomy in shorter operation time by 30 minutes and lower pain scores on the visual analogue scale at 24 hours after surgery.

It is important to examine the merits of different types of hysterectomy in real-world situations outside the arena of randomized controlled trials. In this respect, Juha Mäkinen reported on the outcomes of 10,110 unselected prospective cases of hysterectomy performed by more than 100 gynecologists across 58 hospitals in Finland. There were 5,875

(58.1%) cases of abdominal hysterectomy, 1,801 (17.8%) cases of vaginal hysterectomy, and 2,434 (24.1%) cases of laparoscopic hysterectomy. Vaginal hysterectomy and abdominal hysterectomy were similar in operation duration (86 minutes), length of hospital stay (6 days), blood loss (340 ml), rate of visceral injuries (<1%), and recuperation time (34 days). In comparison to vaginal and abdominal hysterectomy, laparoscopic hysterectomy had a longer operation time (124 minutes), higher rate of visceral injuries (2.8%), shorter length of hospital stay (3.4 days) and recuperation time (21.5 days), and less blood loss (262 ml).

Evidence has shown that the complication rates of laparoscopic hysterectomy decreases with increasing experience of surgeons. An analysis of the Danish national database for hysterectomy which included 51,141 cases reported that, in comparison to vaginal hysterectomy without prolapse, the relative risk of major complications of laparoscopic hysterectomy reduced from 0.96 between 2004 and 2009 to 0.72 between 2010 and 2015. Laparoscopic hysterectomy, however, had a higher risk of minor complications and the trend remained unchanged over the two study periods. The overall complication rates were 19.9% for abdominal hysterectomy, 16.2% for laparoscopic hysterectomy, and 12.9% for vaginal hysterectomy without prolapse.

It is apparent that, for optimal overall clinical outcomes, the best method of hysterectomy for an indication suitable for any of the three surgical approaches is vaginal hysterectomy, followed by laparoscopic hysterectomy and, as a last resort, abdominal hysterectomy.

Indications and Contraindications of Laparoscopic Hysterectomy

Indications

Laparoscopy is a mode of surgery and is not specifically meant for hysterectomy. Laparoscopic hysterectomy is indicated only when a patient is suffering from a uterine condition for which hysterectomy is curative. It is also indicated specifically when vaginal hysterectomy, which is the most efficient mode of surgery, is contraindicated due to pelvic adhesions or endometriosis, a large uterine dimension which limits vaginal access to the upper uterine pedicles, or the need for concomitant ovarian surgery, such as ovarian cystectomy or salpingo-oophorectomy.

Contraindications

Laparoscopic hysterectomy has been shown to be technically feasible for almost all indications of hysterectomy. There are several relative contraindications for laparoscopic hysterectomy based on demands of technical and surgical skill, as well as the surgeon's and patient's level of acceptance of risk of complications. These relative contraindications can be divided into contraindications for laparoscopy as listed in Chapter 6 and contraindications from uterine conditions including:

— Cervical malignancy that warrants a radical hysterectomy,
— Large uterine leiomyomata or uterine adenomyoma that obstructs the lower abdomen,
— Increased uterine width greater than 10 cm, and
— Lateral or lower uterine segment fibroids over 5 cm.

Intraoperative Patient Preparation

Optimal preparation of a patient during surgery is important to achieve the best outcomes for patient safety and surgery. The following steps are not exhaustive but critically important:

— General anesthesia with intubation and mechanical ventilation, continuous cardiopulmonary function monitoring, venous infusion access, and good muscle relaxation.
— Patient positioning: dorsal supine and lithotomy position with the legs rested on Lloyd-Davis or booth-trap stirrups. The buttocks are adjusted to a position that just overhangs the end of the operating table to facilitate the maneuver of uterine manipulators.
— The abdominal skin is coated with antiseptic from the costal margins to the mid-thigh level, there is perineum and vagina cleansing are cleaned with antiseptic solution, and appropriate surgical drapes are applied.
— The urinary bladder is emptied via transurethral catheterization.
— The uterine cervix is dilated and an appropriate intrauterine manipulator is inserted. An assistant sits at the bottom end of the table to manipulate the position of the uterus during surgery.
— Where a steep Trendelenburg tilt is anticipated, shoulder holders or pads may be placed to prevent cephalic slipping of the patient.

Insufflation System

The most widely used insufflation system to create and maintain pneumoperitoneum is an automated electronic controlled pump with adjustable gas flow pressure and flow rate. These parameters are prominently displayed on the front panel of the insufflator. A variety of designs on the flow system allows intra-abdominal gas to be evacuated on one channel, while a separate channel insufflates the gas at a high flow rate to maintain adequate pneumoperitoneum for operative maneuvers.

At the outset of surgery, the predetermined target insufflation pressure is set and gas flow is turned on to determine the unobstructed flow pressure with a Veress needle held in free air. The Veress needle is then turned to a closed state to observe a rise in flow pressure. This is to confirm that the flow system does not have a leakage or any faults.

Pneumoperitoneum Creation and Trocar Insertion

There are no less than 30 different primary trocar insertion techniques described for laparoscopic surgery. Despite the large number of gynecologic and non-gynecologic laparoscopic surgeries over the last 30 years, good quality clinical research on the merits of each method remains sparse. Of great clinical significance are good data on the rate of failure in gaining access into the abdominal cavity and incidence of major complications associated with different methods of trocar entry. Fatal complications from trocar injuries are extremely rare. The most commonly reported causes of fatality were vascular injuries in more than 80% and bowel injuries in the remaining 20% of cases. Although the reported overall incidence of major vascular injuries is less than 1% and bowel injuries less than 0.5%, the absolute number of cases suffering these injuries is large because of the high prevalence rate of laparoscopic surgeries.

These issues were examined in a number of Cochrane systematic reviews, with the most recent publication in 2019. Twenty-five different methods of trocar insertion were compared for incidence of major complications involving (i) mortality, (ii) vascular injury to major intra-abdominal and anterior abdominal wall vessels, (iii) visceral injuries involving the bladder and bowels, (iv) solid organ injury, and (v) gas embolism. Of the 57 randomized controlled trials involving 9,865 patients in the review, there was no evidence of any difference in incidence of major complications between the methods of trocar insertion. Limited data on comparison of the Veress needle method against direct trocar entry suggested that the rate of failure of trocar insertion was lower for direct trocar entry (1.3% versus 6.4%). Whether one method of trocar insertion is superior to others remains unknown for subsets of patients at high risk of major complications. In addition, the failure rate of trocar insertion in patients with previous abdominal surgeries and patients with high body mass index, compared to the general population, is unknown.

There are three basic methods of creating pneumoperitoneum and inserting the primary trocar:

Closed Method

This was the first described method of creating pneumoperitoneum and it is still widely practiced, predominantly among gynecologists. It involves inserting a needle into the peritoneal cavity for CO_2 infusion, followed by blind insertion of a cannula on a sharp trocar.

Veress needle

The Veress needle is a cannula of approximately 2 mm in diameter with a sharp beveled cutting end. The cannula houses an inner spring-loaded stylet that has the blunt end slightly protruding out of the beveled end of the cannula. On meeting tissue resistance during insertion, the stylet retracts to allow the sharp beveled cannula to pierce the tissue. Once the cannula enters the free peritoneal cavity, the spring-loaded stylet emerges to occlude the sharp cannula and avoid injury to other structures. The Veress needle is either 120 mm or 150 mm in length and can be for single use or reusable.

Primary port for trocar and cannula

A basic reusable trocar is a hollow metal pen-like instrument with a triangular tapering terminal that ends in a sharp point. Close to the tapering end is a small fenestration in communication with the central hollow. The opposite terminal end of the trocar is a cap on which hand pressure is applied during insertion. The trocar carries an outer cannula or sheath through which instruments can be introduced. The entire structure is 11 mm in diameter.

Disposable trocars come in a variety of designs, with the sharp end in a conical rather than triangular shape. Some trocars are mounted with a camera for direct visualization of the tissue plane during maneuvers to advance the trocar into the peritoneal cavity.

Technique of umbilical approach

The umbilical approach is the most common mode of creating pneumoperitoneum (Figure 7.1). An alternative approach from the Palmar's point is recommended in cases of suspected lower abdominal adhesions from previous laparotomies.

In the umbilical approach, the patient is put in a supine neutral position and the surgeon stands on the patient's left-hand side. A vertical skin incision of 11 mm is made at the midline position over the umbilical collar and hood, avoiding the umbilical tip (Figure 7.2, Panel (a)). Attention is needed to avoid making a full-thickness incision of the abdominal wall, which is more likely to happen inadvertently in slim and underweight women. The abdominal wall below the umbilicus is lifted vertically. The tip of a Veress

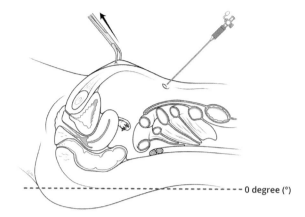

Figure 7.1 ■ An illustration of a patient in a neutral supine position with the lower limbs put in the Lloyd-Davis position.

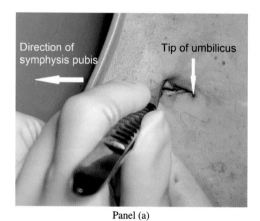

Figure 7.2 ■ Panel (a) is a surgical photograph showing a vertical incision of 11 mm over the umbilical hood in full thickness to divide the umbilical collar. Panel (b) shows the technique of inserting a Veress needle.

needle is placed in the umbilical incision and the needle is pushed into the peritoneal cavity in a controlled manner. The needle should be in a 45° inclination targeting the center of the plane of the pelvic inlet and the direction maintained at the midline to avoid deviating from the subumbilical triangle marking on the abdomen (Figure 7.2, Panel (b)). A distinct sensation of tissue giving way will be felt twice as the needle pierces through the rectus sheath and the peritoneum.

Wiggling the Veress needle to confirm its position in the free abdominal cavity should strictly be disallowed as the needle my lacerate parts of the bowel or vascular structures. The position of the tip of the Veress needle in the peritoneal cavity can be tested by the instillation of clear saline solution injected through the needle, or by dropping level of a saline drop at the top of the needle hub. Once the insufflation starts, the flow pressure should not exceed 8 mmHg. Insufflation is continued until a flow pressure of 25 mmHg is reached. It has been shown that this pressure is associated with splinting of the abdominal wall with only a small downward displacement of the umbilicus into the abdominal cavity on encountering the thrusting force during insertion of the trocar. The resulting large distance between the anterior abdominal wall and the underlying intra-abdominal structures and major vessels reduces the risk of trocar-related injuries to intra-abdominal and retro-peritoneal structures. The Veress needle is withdrawn and the patient is ready for insertion of the trocar.

If Veress insertion is unsuccessful in gaining access to the free peritoneal cavity, a second attempt can be done. If it fails again, I recommend switching to the open method of trocar insertion.

Insertion of primary trocar

With the surgeon's hand in a palm up position, the shaft of the trocar is held between the index and middle fingers. The cap of the trocar is next to the thenar eminence. The trocar is firmly gripped in this position with the thenar eminence covering the cap (Figure 7.3) and inserted through the umbilical incision vertically. The force of trocar insertion should be in controlled, forward-twisting movements instead of a forceful thrust. Once in the abdominal cavity, a gush of gas through the cap will be heard. The gas leak from the cap is stopped by moving the right thumb over it. With the trocar held steady by the cap, the cannula is pushed a small distance further into abdominal cavity to ensure that its tip is entirely intraperitoneal before the trocar is removed.

Gas insufflation

The gas insufflation tube is connected to the cannula for maintenance of pneumoperitoneum.

— A laparoscope, with the video camera mounted, is then introduced through the cannula for intra-abdominal inspection.

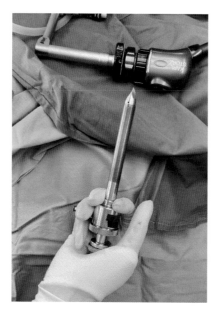

Figure 7.3 ■ A surgical photograph showing the correct handling of the primary trocar in preparation for insertion into the peritoneal cavity.

Open Method

The most common open method of pneumoperitoneum creation is the Hasson method described in 1970. It involves making a small periumbilical incision into the abdominal cavity in the form of a mini laparotomy. A blunt end trocar is then placed in the opening under direct vision, as compared to the blind insertion in the closed method described above. The cannula is secured for gas insufflation and instrument introduction.

Technique

A semi-lunar or midline skin incision is made over the hood of the umbilicus. The dermis, not skin, is held up with two artery forceps. The subcutaneous tissues are further dissected to reveal the linea alba, which is then grasped and lifted with two artery forceps and incised with a scalpel. The preperitoneal tissues are cleared from peritoneum which is then picked up with artery forceps and incised with a sharp scalpel carefully to enter the peritoneal cavity. A small S-retractor is inserted into the abdominal cavity to retract the incision laterally so that a right and left lateral sutures can be placed at the sides of the laparotomy aperture to include the peritoneal edge and the lineal alba. A blunt Hasson trocar is placed through the aperture and the two side sutures are secured to the thread holders on the trocar to maintain air tightness and to prevent the trocar from slipping out of the incision. The obturator is removed and the gas insufflation tubing is connected.

Direct Trocar Entry Method

This is a closed method in which the sharp trocar is inserted into the abdominal cavity without prior needle insufflation of gas. It replaces two blinded insertions of a Veress needle and trocar with a single blinded trocar insertion.

Technique

The umbilicus is held and pulled up with a pair of toothed forceps. A vertical incision cuts through the full thickness of skin across the entire diameter of the umbilicus. Two towel clips are applied to both sides of the incision. The clip should include the entire thickness of incision and the peripheral skin to hold the umbilicus strongly. The clips are pulled vertically upward as high as possible to elevate the anterior abdominal wall away from the intra-abdominal structures and aorta. The trocar is then pushed through the incision vertically without deviation. A laparoscope is introduced to confirm successful peritoneal access before commencing gas insufflation.

Second and Third Trocar Insertions

The number of secondary trocars for laparoscopic hysterectomy depends on the surgeon's preference over the types and number of instruments needed. The most important determinants in selecting the locations for operative trocars are proficiency of surgical maneuvers and risk of complications based on anatomical considerations. The exact location is based on the balance between ease of access to targeted pedicles and potential clashes between instruments in the camera port and the second port (Figure 7.4).

Using an operative camera laparoscope that has a channel for operative instruments, I need only one second trocar for LAVH. In this procedure, as surgical maneuvers target the upper pedicles at the lateral borders of the uterus, the best position for the second trocar is at the midline between the umbilicus and the pubic symphysis (Figure 7.5).

Once the appropriate location has been determined, a 5 mm skin incision is made with a sharp scalpel. The 5 mm trocar is inserted under direct vision from a laparoscope. The vertical controlled forward-twisting maneuver of insertion is the same as the description for insertion of the primary trocar. Once the tip of the trocar presses immediately on the peritoneum (Figure 7.6), the direction of the trocar can be adjusted to point into parts of the peritoneal cavity that are free from viscera and solid organ. The trocar is finally pushed to pierce the peritoneum. Once the canula is confirmed to be intraperitoneal, the trocar is removed and the operative instrument is introduced through the canula.

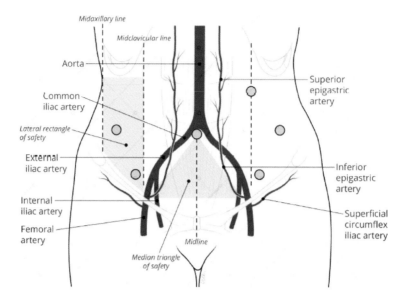

Figure 7.4 ■ An illustration of possible locations on the anterior abdominal wall for the placement of instrument ports.

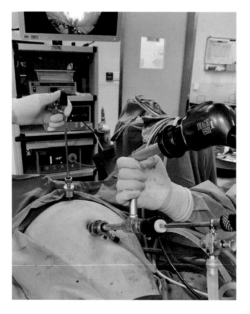

Figure 7.5 ■ A surgical photograph showing the positions of primary and second ports in a case of laparoscopy-assisted vaginal hysterectomy.

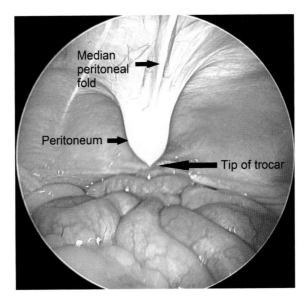

Figure 7.6 ■ A surgical photograph showing the insertion of a suprapubic trocar under direct vision.

Hysterectomy Procedures

Division of Round Ligaments

The uterus is pushed up into the mid-pelvic cavity and deviated toward the left-hand side by the assistant controlling the uterine manipulator. The right round ligament is seen as a taut cord. A pair of short Manhe's forceps in the second port is used to grasp the round ligament at the midpoint between the cornua of the uterus and the internal inguinal ring. A gentle upward lifting of the ligament will show its entire thickness in the broad ligament, with the Sampson artery running inferior and parallel to the ligament. A pair of bipolar diathermy forceps in the operative channel of the laparoscope is applied perpendicularly to the entire thickness of the round ligament and Sampson artery. These structures are cauterized and divided (Figure 7.7).

The broad ligament is opened and divided using monopolar scissors toward the vesicouterine space anteriorly. Laterally, the broad ligament is opened parallel to the infundibulopelvic ligament (Figure 7.8).

With the uterus stabilized in the left-sided deviation, the cut edge of the medial leaf of the left right broad ligament is held taut by upward lifting with a pair of Manhes' forceps, and the retroperitoneal space is opened with the loose areolar tissues pushed

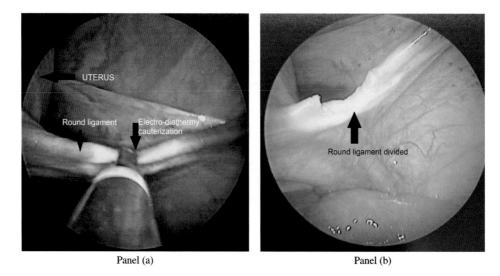

Panel (a)   Panel (b)

Figure 7.7 ■ Surgical photographs showing cauterization (Panel (a)) and division (Panel (b)) of the round ligament.

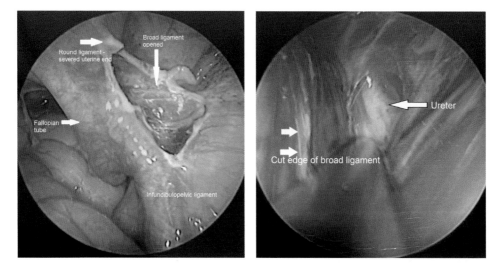

Figure 7.8 ■ A surgical photograph showing the opening of the lateral broad ligament parallel to the infundibulopelvic ligament.

away to show the nearly transparent posterior leave of the broad ligament. The ureter can often easily be seen a distance inferior to the infundibulopelvic ligament (Figure 7.8).

A similar procedure is performed on the contralateral round ligament with the uterus deviated toward the right-hand side. More often than not, the sigmoid colon is loosely attached to the left round ligament by loose and flimsy fibrous tissue sheets. The sheets should be released to mobilize the colon away from the uterine appendages.

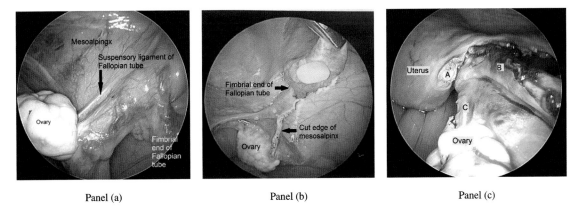

Panel (a)   Panel (b)   Panel (c)

Figure 7.9 ■ Panel (a) is a surgical photograph showing the suspensory ligament of the Fallopian tube being held in a taut position. Panel (b) shows that the Fallopian tube has been mobilized from the mesosalpinx attachment. Panel (c) shows the Fallopian tube stump.

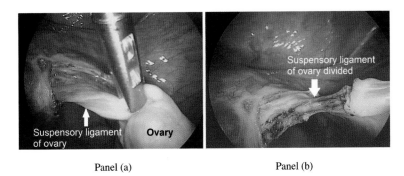

Panel (a)   Panel (b)

Figure 7.10 ■ Surgical photographs showing cauterization and division of an ovarian ligament.

Division of Mesosalpinx

The ampulla of the Fallopian tube is grasped with a pair of Manhe's forceps and the tube is lifted upward and straightened. The mesosalpinx is thus straightened and kept taut (Figure 7.9, Panels (a) and (b)). The suspensory ligament of the fimbria to the ovary is cauterized and divided. The division of the remaining part of the mesosalpinx is performed along the inferior border of the Fallopian tube toward its junction with the uterus. Panel (c) of Figure 7.9 shows a Fallopian tube that has been excised.

Division of the Ovarian Ligaments

The ovary is grasped with Manhe's forceps and gently retracted from the uterus. The anastomotic utero-ovarian vessels are seen superior to the ovarian suspensory ligament (Figure 7.10, Panel (a)). The vessels are sealed with electrocautery at a point approximately 1 cm away from the uterus and divided using sharp scissors. At this point, the ovarian suspensory ligament is cauterized and divided and the ovary is mobilized (Figure 7.10, Panel (b)).

Division of Infundibulopelvic Ligaments for Hysterectomy with Removal of the Ovary

After division of the round ligament, the superior border of the broad ligament is incised parallel to the infundibulopelvic ligament to a distance 1 to 2 cm away from the cephalic pole of the ovary. The medial leaf of the broad ligament is held taut and the retroperitoneal space is opened as described above to identify the ureter (Figure 7.8). The full thickness of the infundibulopelvic ligament can now be identified. A window is made on the clear leaf of the broad ligament inferior to the ligament. Bipolar electrodiathermy forceps are applied across the skeletonized infundibulopelvic ligament, which is then divided after complete sealing with electrodiathermy cauterization (Figure 7.11, Panel (a)). The severed uterine portion of the infundibulopelvic ligament is mobilized toward the uterus until the insertion of the cervical portion of the uterosacral ligament to the uterus (Figure 7.11, Panels (b) and (c)).

Opening of the Vesicouterine Space

The incised edge of the anterior broad ligament at the lateral border of the cervix is held taut with Manhe's forceps and the vesicouterine space is tunneled by blunt dissection with a probe or the tip of monopolar diathermy scissors, starting from the lateral border and progressing toward the midline. The overlying peritoneum is then incised (Figure 7.12). Once the entire vesicouterine peritoneum has been incised, the loose fatty

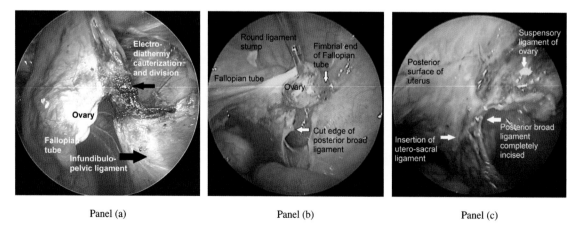

| Panel (a) | Panel (b) | Panel (c) |

Figure 7.11 ■ Panel (a): A surgical photograph showing cauterization of the infundibulopelvic ligament. Panels (b) and (c) show the division of the broad ligament to the uterine border.

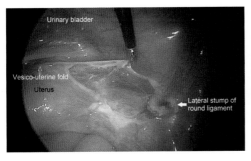
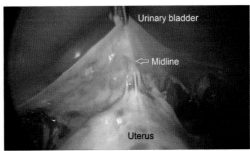

Panel (a)   Panel (b)

Figure 7.12 ■ The vesicouterine space is opened from the lateral borders toward the midline (Panel (a)) and then incised at the midline (Panel (b)).

tissue in the vesicouterine space is pushed downwards and anteriorly. The urinary bladder base is then pushed away from the cervix. Superficial diathermy cauterization may be necessary to arrest bleeding.

Surgical Variation According to Different Types of Laparoscopic Hysterectomy

For Laparoscopy-assisted Vaginal Hysterectomy

The laparoscopic procedure for LAVH is complete once the superior pedicles of hysterectomy are divided. The remainder of the hysterectomy is accomplished transvaginally as described in Chapter 5 on vaginal hysterectomy.

For Laparoscopic Hysterectomy

Laparoscopic hysterectomy includes complete division of the superior uterine pedicles as well as the uterine vessels. In addition to dividing the superior uterine pedicles and vesicouterine space, the posterior cervicovaginal peritoneum is opened.

Opening of posterior cervicovaginal peritoneum

The uterus is elevated in the cranial direction, pointing anteriorly. The uterorectal fold of the peritoneum is held up at the midline position close to the inferior border of the cervix and incised with a pair of scissors. The uterus is then slightly deviated toward the contralateral side while the peritoneal incision is extended toward the uterosacral ligament.

Sealing and dividing the uterine vessels

The uterus is manipulated cranially, pointing anteriorly, and maintained in a slight deviation toward the contralateral side with the uterine manipulator and the traction at the uterine stump of the round ligament. The loose tissue in the lateral parametrium is cleared with gentle pushing actions using the slightly opened tip of a pair of dissecting scissors to show the uterine vessels at the lateral border of the uterus. The ureter position is inspected and uterine vessels are electrocauterized immediately lateral to the uterus, commencing from the ascending branch (Figure 7.13).

Colpotomy for removal of the uterus and closure of the vaginal vault is completed via a transvaginal route as in vaginal hysterectomy.

For Total Laparoscopic Hysterectomy

As the definition of TLH includes division of all pedicles to produce a free uterus in the peritoneal cavity, the instrumentation requires second and third trocar ports. Apart from the primary trocar port at the umbilicus, the other two 5 mm ports are sited within the lateral zones of safety at the lower abdomen, typically lateral to the rectus muscles at the level just above the anterior superior iliac spines (Figure 7.4). The ports are inserted under

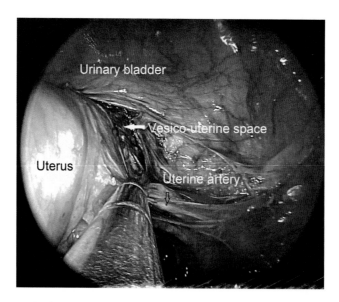

Figure 7.13 ■ A surgical photograph showing the position of cauterization and division of the uterine artery.

direct vision. A uterine manipulator, such as a colpotomizer with a vaginal occlusion balloon, is essential for completion of uterine amputation laparoscopically.

Placement of the uterine manipulator

— The anterior lip of cervix is held with a tenaculum, the length of the uterine cavity is measured with a uterine sound, and the width of the cervix is measured with a cervical sizer.
— A uterine manipulation tip of equal length to the uterine cavity and a Koh-efficient colpotomizer cup of equal size to the cervix are selected (Figure 7.14, Panel (a)). The uterine tip is attached securely to the end of an Advincular Arch uterine manipulator using a twist-and-push maneuver. The uterine balloon catheter and uterine cavity

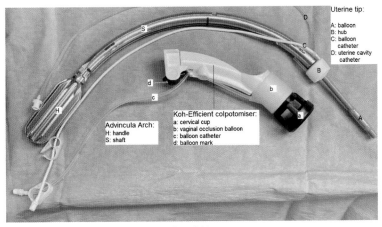

Panel (a)

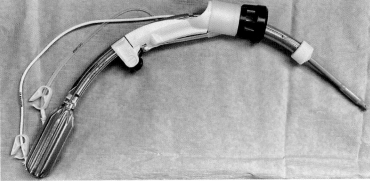

Panel (b)

Figure 7.14 ■ These photographs show a uterine manipulator (Adventula Arch) and a Koh colpotomizer (Panel (a)), and the assembly of the manipulator before insertion into the uterine cavity (Panel (b)).

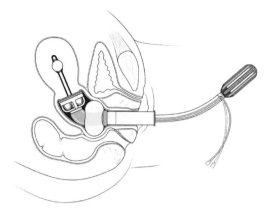

Figure 7.15 ■ A sketch illustrating the setup of a uterine manipulator and colpotomizer.

insufflation catheter are placed in the groove at the side of the shaft of the Advicular Arch. The Koh-efficient colpotomizer is placed onto the Advincular Arch (Figure 7.14, Panel (b) and Figure 7.15).

— The cervix is dilated to size Hegar-8.
— The uterine tip on the assembled Advincular Arch is introduced into the uterine cavity through the cervical os until the hub of the tip is flushed with the cervix. The uterine balloon is insufflated with 6 ml of sterile water to secure it in position.
— The tenaculum is removed and the colpotomizer is advanced into the vagina, taking care not to traumatize the mucosa of the introitus and vagina.
— The colpotomizer is pushed onto the cervix until the cervical cup locks onto the hub of the uterine tip. After confirming the correct placement of the colpotomizer cup on the cervix by digital palpation, the balloon mark of the colpotomizer is pressed onto the Advincular Arch manipulator to stabilize the cup.
— The vaginal pneumo-occluder is insufflated with 60 ml of saline.

Surgery of the upper uterine pedicles

The upper uterine pedicles are managed as described above. It is also necessary to place an appropriate uterine manipulator with a peumo-occluder through the vagina to maintain pneumoperitoneum for colpotomy and removal of the uterus through the vagina.

Colpotomy

The cap of the uterine manipulator used in TLH would help with identifying the vaginal fornix when the uterus is pushed cranially. Adequate opening of the vesicouterine space to the level just below the fornix is necessary (Figure 7.16).

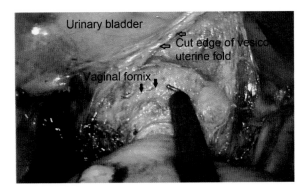

Figure 7.16 ■ A surgical photograph showing the identification of colpotomizer over the anterior vaginal fornix.

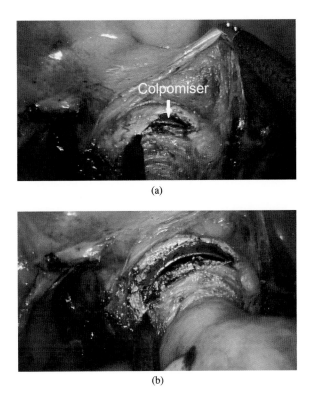

Figure 7.17 ■ Surgical photographs showing the colpotomy procedure.

The cervical portion of the transverse and uterosacral ligaments are pushed laterally with a probe. Colpotomy is performed from the midline of the anterior fornix and extended lateroposteriorly to complete the circumferential incision (Figure 7.17). The uterus is retrieved transvaginally. Uterine morcellation may be necessary if the uterus volume is too large to be removed in one piece. This is achieved by coring the central part of the uterus with a sharp scalpel.

Repair of the vaginal vault

Vaginal balloon is inflated to maintain pneumoperitoneum. The right and left lateral vaginal angles are secured with sutures incorporating the uterosacral ligaments, transverse ligaments, and posterior vaginal wall as described in the procedure for McCall culdoplasty. The remaining part of the vaginal vault is closed in full thickness with interrupted sutures.

Recent reports of a significant incidence of vaginal vault dehiscence following TLH has prompted some to advocate transvaginal closure of vaginal vault as described for LAVH in Chapter 5.

Completion of Laparoscopy

Hemostasis is inspected and secured, peritoneal washing is performed, pneumoperitoneam gas is expelled, and trocars are removed. Finally, the skin incision is closed with 3-O Vicryl sutures.

References

Aarts JWM, Nieboer TE, Johnson N, *et al.* (2015) Surgical approach to hysterectomy for benign gynaecological disease. *Cochrane Database Syst Rev* **8**: CD003677. DOI:10.1002/14651858. CD003677.pub5.

Ahmad G, Baker J, Finnerty J, *et al.* (2019) Laparoscopic entry techniques. *Cochrane Database Syst Rev* **1**: CD006583.

Ala-Nissilä S, Laurikainen E, Mäkinen J, *et al.* (2019) Vaginal cuff dehiscence is observed in a higher rate after total laparoscopic hysterectomy compared with other types of hysterectomy. *Acta Obstet Gynecol Scand* **98**: 44–50.

Domingo S, Pellicer A. (2009) Overview of current trends in hysterectomy. *Expert Rev of Obstet Gynecol* **4**(6): 673–685.

Garry R, Fountain J, Mason S, *et al.* (2004) The eVALuate study: two parallel randomised trials, one comparing laparoscopic with abdominal hysterectomy, the other comparing laparoscopic with vaginal hysterectomy. *BMJ* **328**(7432): 129–133.

Istre O, Snejbjerg D. (2018) Complication rate of laparoscopic hysterectomies in Denmark, 2011–2016. *JSLS* **22**: e2017.00078

Lee SH, Oh SR, Cho YJ, *et al.* (2019) Comparison of vaginal hysterectomy and laparoscopic hysterectomy: a systematic review and meta-analysis. *BMC Women's Health* **19**: 83

Loring M, Morris SN, Isaacson KB. (2015) Minimally invasive specialists and rates of laparoscopic hysterectomy. *JSLS* **19**: e2014.00221

Madhvani K, Curnow T, Carpenter T. (2019) Route of hysterectomy: a retrospective, cohort study in English NHS Hospitals from 2011 to 2017. *BJOG* **126**: 795–802.

NICE. Interventional procedure overview of laparoscopic hysterectomy. National Institute for Clinical Excellence, UK 2004; 1–16.

Reich H. (2007) Total laparoscopic hysterectomy: indications, techniques and outcomes. *Curr Opin Obstet Gynecol* **19**: 337–344.

Sandberg EM, Twijnstra ARH, Driessen SRC, *et al.* (2017) Total laparoscopic hysterectomy versus vaginal hysterectomy: a systematic review and meta-analysis. *J Minim Invasive Gynecol* **24**(2): 206–217.e22. doi: 10.1016/j.jmig.2016.10.020. Epub 2016 Nov 17. PMID: 27867051.

Schmitt JJ, Leon DAC, Occhino JA, *et al.* (2017) Determining optimal route of hysterectomy for benign indications: clinical decision tree algorithm. *Obstet Gynecol* **129**(1): 130–138.

Settnes A, Moeller C, Topsoee MF, *et al.* (2020) Complications after benign hysterectomy, according to procedure: a population-based prospective cohort study from the DANISH hysterectomy database, 2004–2015*BJOG* **127**: 1269–1279.

Thurston J, Murji A, Scattolon S, *et al.* (2019) Hysterectomy for benign gynaecologic indications. *J Obstet Gynaecol Can* **41**(4): 543–557. doi: 10.1016/j.jogc.2018.12.006. PMID: 30879487.

8

Perioperative Care

Surgery is often seen as a dramatic, heroic performance and a technical feat. Not surprisingly, the operation room has traditionally been termed a theater. What matters, however, is the outcome of the patient from the surgical procedure.

Surgical technique defines surgery, but the patient's outcome is determined by a myriad of factors, including the patient's constitution, comorbidity, and environment, which require optimal perioperative care with appropriate contributions possibly from physicians of multiple disciplines. The aim of this chapter is to highlight the role of a surgeon in perioperative care for enhanced recovery from hysterectomy, which involves:

a.   Identification of significant conditions requiring care from other specialists;
b.   Optimizing the risk profile of patients;
c.   Taking measures to optimize surgical recovery; and
d.   Early identification and prompt institution of remedy for surgical complications.

Preoperative Care

The Decision on Hysterectomy

Perioperative care begins with the surgeon's and patient's decision to undertake hysterectomy. Three key responsibilities of a surgeon in this respect are:

Confirmation of diagnosis

It is the ultimate role of the surgeon to establish that the diagnosis of the woman's condition for which the consultation is sought is accurate. This is the basis for recommending hysterectomy as the remedy for the condition. A detailed discussion of indications of hysterectomy has been presented in Chapter 1.

Selecting the type of hysterectomy

The merits and shortcomings of each type of hysterectomy have been discussed in earlier descriptions of individual types of hysterectomy. The surgeon must put the patient's interests before his own preference and technical expertise when advising the patient on the best method of hysterectomy for her condition. If the best type of hysterectomy happens to be beyond one's technical skillset, one should inform the patient accordingly and discuss the option of referring her to another surgeon who can deliver the most appropriate type of hysterectomy.

Informed consent

The taking of informed consent begins with informing the patient of the diagnosis of her condition and a succinct discussion and appraisal of merits and shortcomings of available legitimate treatment methods. The patient must be given enough time to reach a firm decision on her choice of treatment option. If hysterectomy is opted, a signed written consent with appropriate witness is necessary.

Preoperative Assessment of the Patient

Surgery is a risky endeavor for the surgeon and patient. The famous surgeon, Dr Hermann Johannes Pfannenstiel, died from staphylococcus aureus infection after sustaining a finger needle-stick injury during an operation on a woman with tubo-ovarian abscess. Some communicable diseases can harm surgical team members, paramedical personnel, or fellow patients. There should be active screening of prevalent communicable diseases in the community so that appropriate preventive measures against cross-infection during delivery of healthcare can be instituted. Prevalent contemporary infectious conditions include human immunodeficiency virus infection, hepatitis virus B and C infection, and methicillin-resistant staphylococcus aureus infection.

The other primary objective of preoperative examination is to understand the risk profile of the patient which influences the safety of surgery on her. Many conditions in the risk profile are amenable to modification through appropriate interventions.

Nutrition

Malnutrition is uncommon in Singapore and other economically well-to-do countries except in women with coexisting medical conditions such as cancer, malabsorption from intestinal disorders, chronic ill health, and psychiatric diseases. Independent of associated medical conditions, malnutrition adversely affects physiological responses to surgery with compromises on safety of surgery and mortality rate. It also delays surgical wound healing.

Nutritional insufficiency may be inconspicuous and identifiable only through assays of serum albumin level.

Obesity

Obesity is commonly associated with hypertension, diabetes mellitus, and obstructive sleep apnea. It is an independent high-risk factor for increased incidence of prolonged surgical duration, blood loss and blood transfusion, respiratory and urinary tract infections, surgical infections, wound dehiscence, thromboembolism, and mortality.

Appropriate time must be given for the patient to optimize her body weight before hysterectomy.

Cigarette smoking

Chronic cigarette smokers are prone to obstructive airway disorders and thromboembolic phenomena. Patients are advised to stop smoking for four to eight weeks before admission to hospital for hysterectomy.

Comorbid medical conditions

Both the uterine pathology and chronological age profile of the woman are commonly associated with a number of comorbidities. Not uncommonly, multiple comorbidities are found on the same patient, such as:

o   Anemia
o   Hypertension
o   Ischemic heart disease
o   Diabetes mellitus and endocrinopathy
o   Renal diseases
o   Thromboembolism

Each of these comorbidities independently increases perioperative life-threatening complications such as acute coronary events or myocardial infarction, cerebrovascular accidents, pulmonary embolism, and acute renal failure. It is the surgeon's duty to take necessary measures to prevent the infamous situation where "a patient underwent a successful surgery but died of complications".

On detecting any of these comorbidities, the surgeon should refer the patient to appropriate physicians for optimization of disease control and continual postoperative management. The additional risk of complications associated with the comorbidity must be clearly communicated to the patient.

Preoperative Preparation of the Uterus

Symptomatic uterine fibroids are the most common cause of hysterectomy for benign pathology. It is not uncommon for the size of the uterus to be hugely enlarged by tumors. An estimated absolute uterine volume of 500 ml or more from ultrasonographic scanning is an independent predictor of major intraoperative complications for all types of hysterectomy, including severe hemorrhage, ureteric and urinary bladder injuries, bowel injuries, and prolonged duration of operation time. It is also a risk factor for postoperative infection and sepsis.

Gonadotropin-releasing hormone agonists (GnRHa), by downregulating ovarian estrogen secretion, have been shown to reduce the volume of uterine fibroids by 50% within 3 months of treatment. Available evidence indicates that preoperative treatment with GnRHa increases the number of women suitable for vaginal hysterectomy and reduces the number of women who require a vertical incision in abdominal hysterectomy. There is also a significant reduction in major intraoperative complications during hysterectomy. The associated amenorrhea during the treatment period has also been shown to improve patients' preoperative hemoglobin and hematocrit levels. However, the cost effectiveness of this line of treatment for all hysterectomy performed for symptomatic uterine fibroids remains unproven. Together with adverse effects, the use of preoperative GnRHa is best considered an individualized treatment guided by the absolute volume of the uterus and the choice of the patient.

Intraoperative Care

Antibiotic Prophylaxis

Surgery-related infection is a significant complication that delays patients' recovery and increases the length of hospital stay or chances of readmission after initial discharge.

In hysterectomy, the common sources of microorganisms are the vagina, gut, and skin. There is good evidence to show that preoperative prophylaxis with a broad-spectrum antibiotic reduces perioperative infection following hysterectomy. The current recommended choice of antimicrobial medication is a single dose of amoxicillin-clavulanic acid 1.2 g or cehazolin 2 g administered intravenously 60 minutes before skin incision. If hypersensitivity to penicillin is present, the combination of clindamycin 600 mg diluted in 100 ml of 0.9% sodium chloride infused over 20 minutes intravenously and gentamicin 80 mg intravenously are preferred.

Antithrombotic Measures

Mortality from hysterectomy is rare. A 2015 report based on a retrospective study of 20,496 hysterectomies in the US showed that the death rate from women who developed venous thromboembolism (VTE) was 9 times higher compared to those who did not have VTE (0.91% versus 0.1%). The report revealed that VTE, overall, was not rare. The incidence was 0.53%, consisting of deep vein thrombosis (0.20%), pulmonary embolism (0.27%), and concurrent deep vein thrombosis and pulmonary embolism (0.06%). Nonfatal VTE is often associated with significant long-term sequelae.

Lower limb compression stockings and pneumatic lower limb compression are effective preventive measures against VTE from venous stasis. These measures should begin from the onset of surgery and to be continued postoperatively until the patient is able to ambulate fully.

Body Fluid Management

Close collaboration b1etween the surgeon and anesthesiologist is essential for maintaining optimal body fluid balance and body temperature. Blood loss may lead to hypovolemia which comprises cardiovascular hemodynamics. Fluid overload increases the risk of respiratory compromises and peripheral edema delays surgical wound healing.

Body Temperature Management

General anesthesia lowers body temperature by disturbing the body's physiological thermoregulatory response to hypothermia. It also dampens the autonomic responses of thermoregulation. The loss of these functions is particularly evident in patients who are unable to elicit voluntary actions to raise their body temperature. Consequently, hypothermia is a common phenomenon in patients during surgery.

It is recommended that the patient's intraoperative body temperature is maintained at >36°C. Mild hypothermia (35°C –36°C) is associated with tachycardia and increased oxygen consumption, while more severe hypothermia (33°C to 35°C) can lead to brady-cardia and demonstrable platelet and coagulation cascade dysfunctions which increase surgical blood loss. The postoperative shivering response further stresses the tensile integrity of surgical wounds and increases incidence of wound infection and wound pain.

Measures to maintain the patient's body temperature include:

o Use of prewarmed fluid for infusion and peritoneal washing;
o Use of patient cutaneous warming devices such as cotton blankets and warm water bath blankets; and
o Maintaining optimal ambient temperature in the operating room.

Immediate Postsurgical Care

Immediate Period Following Surgery

Monitoring of vital signs

Surgery is an iatrogenic assault to the physical body. Physiological responses are expected by nature but may be suboptimal to meet the demands of bodily functions. Surgeons should monitor physiological responses so that prompt intervention can be implemented to augment the physiology of nature. While it remains impossible and impractical to investigate all physiological responses, some are critical for life maintenance. These include:

o Cardiovascular function: heart rate and blood pressure, or continuous electrocardiography if indicated.
o Body temperature
o Respiratory function: respiratory rate and oxygen saturation
o Renal function: urinary output

These vital signs are measured hourly during the first 24 hours and 4-hourly on the second day, according to the needs and conditions of the patient.

Pain management

The severity and duration of surgical pain experienced by a patient is influenced by the extent of surgical resection, type of surgical wound, presence of early wound complications such as hematoma, and personal factors that modulate the perception of pain in general. Pain control extends from commencement of surgery to the post-operative period.

Pain control during surgery

Intraoperative pain control is managed by anesthetists. It suffices for surgeons to note the current trend of replacing traditional opioid products with intravenously administered non-opioid medications. Surgeons, however, play an important role in initiating postoperative pain control intraoperatively using local anesthetics.

Local anesthetic infiltration

Local anaesthetic infiltration (LAI) is a simple technique that can be used for laparotomy and laparoscopic wounds. The infiltration is delivered with a gauge-22 needle into the peritoneal, musculofascial, and subdermal tissues along the entire edges of the wound. The volume of infiltration is approximately 1.5 ml per centimeter of the wound. The most widely used local anesthetic for this purpose is bupivacaine (0.25% w/v), which becomes effective within 1 to 3 minutes and the effective duration is between 3 to 4 hours. An alternative anesthetic is ropivacaine.

Continuous wound infusion of local anesthetics

Compared to LIA, which is a one-time wound infiltration with limited duration of pain control, the continuous wound infusion technique allows continual use of local anesthetics for several days. A specific catheter is inserted supraperitoneally with an introducing needle piercing the skin 3 cm lateral to the incision edge. The catheter is connected to an electronic-controlled pump to deliver controlled doses of anesthetic.

Pain control after surgery

Regardless of intraoperative measures, effective pain control remains an important aspect of surgical care. The mean pain score based on the visual analogue scale during the first postoperative hour varies from 6.5 for abdominal hysterectomy to 6 for laparoscopic vaginal hysterectomy and 4.5 for laparoscopic total hysterectomy. The effective pain control regimen typically includes a combination of oral paracetamol 1 g strictly once every 6 hours and celecoxib 200 mg once every 12 hours on the first day, after which it is reduced to once a day from the second day onwards. In the case of laparotomy, additional patient-controlled analgesia of morphine is indicated.

Additional analgesia may be required for some patients. The preferred medication is tramadol 50 mg given at 6- to 8-hourly intervals or codeine 30 mg at 6-hourly intervals. In cases with breakthrough pain on the above management regimen, oral mist morphine of 5 to 10 mg at 4-hourly intervals can be given.

Perioperative nausea and vomiting

At least 40% of patients encounter perioperative nausea and vomiting following hysterectomy, which can be managed with dual antiemetics of intravenously administered dexamethasone 8 mg and ondansetron 4 mg. These antiemetics should be given prophylactically to women with previous history of perioperative nausea and vomiting.

Fluid balance

As surgery induces body fluid loss, intraoperative fluid balance is monitored and managed by anesthetists. The fluid regime is further extended to postoperative care with appropriate modification to maintain homeostasis and hemodynamic and electrolyte balance. In uncomplicated hysterectomy in healthy women, the fluid balance is maintained through simple fluid replacement by taking account of daily physiological requirements and extent of surgical fluid loss. The typical 24-hour fluid replacement is the sum of 1000 ml of fluid and measured volume of fluid loss from urine and surgical drains. This is modified according to clinical signs of hypovolemia which include increased thirst, loss of skin turgor, reduced volume of urine output, hypotension and tachycardia, or fluid overload which may present in peripheral edema or pulmonary edema. Most commonly, the replacing fluid is a crystalloid solution.

In patients who sustain large volumes of fluid and blood loss during surgery or who develop postoperative intestinal ileus, managing the fluid balance becomes more challenging. Additional monitoring of fluid volume balance with a central venous pressure is indicated.

Alimentation

Early alimentation with clear oral fluid should begin early on the day of surgery and progress to full feeds by the end of the day. Soft diet can resume on the second day and progress to a full diet of the patient's choice according to her tolerance of feeds previously.

Antithrombotic management

Pneumatic pressure on the lower limbs should be continued on the first day of surgery while the patient remains bedbound. This is discontinued once she is able to ambulate voluntarily. The use of lower limb passive pressure stockings should continue even after she has been discharged from the hospital. For patients who are assessed to be outside the high-risk category for thromboembolism, the benefit of additional pharmacological anti-coagulation with low-molecular weight heparin is yet to be proven.

Wound management

Surgical wound healing begins from the incision of the skin when platelet activation in hemostasis sets off a coagulation cascade and myriads of cytokine secretion, followed by an inflammatory response. There is an influx of leucocytes and macrophages within the first 24 hours. While neutrophils and lymphocytes are essential in tackling any bacteria present in the wound, macrophages play an integral role in initiating re-epithelialization, granulation formation, and angiogenesis. Re-epithelialization begins from the edge of the wound within the first 24 hours. Keratocytes from the surrounding hair follicles and apocrine gland migrate to fill up the stratum basale layer of the skin and, together with the extracellular matrix material, form the new basement membrane. This is covered by a layer of sterile exudate containing growth factors to promote wound healing. This cellular proliferation phase is accompanied by synthesis of extracellular matrix, fibrinogen, and collagen. The entire process may extend to 4 weeks. Complete wound healing involves a final stage of tissue remodeling where type-3 collagen is replaced by type-1 collagen to return to the original ratio of 4:1 in the skin. The process typically extends to a year or longer. The tensile strength of the wound returns to approximately 60% of that of the original tissue by 4–5 weeks and to 80% by the end of the first year. Primary wound closure, by approximating the wound edges, facilitates many of these processes physically.

The measures of wound management aim to optimize natural wound healing by mitigating the factors that adversely interfere with physiology.

Prevention of local infection

Surgical site infection complicates approximately 10% of abdominal wounds after hysterectomy. Most of these resolve on simple antibiotic treatment, but infection is the most common factor hindering optimal wound healing. Preventive measures for surgical wound infection include:

Preoperative measures such as antiseptic skin prep and antimicrobial prophylaxis before skin incision.

Proper surgical techniques such as avoiding tissue injuries from excessive traction, good hemostasis to prevent wound hematoma, avoiding tissue devitalization from coagulation, minimizing the use of suture material which is a form of foreign body, and applying appropriate wound dressing to create a mechanical barrier to bacterial colonization of the wound. There is no conclusive evidence indicating superiority of one type of surgical dressing over others.

Postoperative measures should include leaving the dressing untouched for up to 48 hours and applying good aseptic technique in changing the dressing when needed. Showering is permitted after 48 hours.

Management of wound exudate

Physiological exudate is an essential part of wound healing. However, overabundant exudates from exaggerated inflammatory response in the wound during the immediate postoperative period may cause skin maceration and delayed wound healing. Appropriate surgical dressing that absorbs the excessive exudate is indicated. Widely available surgical dressings in general operating rooms include sterile gauze and preparations combining layers of fluid absorbing pad and skin adhesive. Some dressings are also impregnated with ionic silver. No one type of surgical dressing is definitively superior to the others.

Nutritional management

Low serum albumin level has been shown to be an independent predictor of surgical wound infection in hysterectomy. Maintaining an adequate calorie and protein intake supplemented by postoperative high doses of vitamin C has been recommended.

Management of chronic illnesses

Obesity, diabetes mellitus, chronic renal failure, and cancer are well-recognized diseases that delay wound healing. Optimal management of these conditions during perioperative periods is critical in promoting wound healing.

Ambulation

Physical activity following surgery, particularly walking, is an important part of functional recovery and is critically important in preventing deep vein thrombosis and pulmonary atelectasis. Patients must receive good pain control as incidence of distressing pain increases by 20% during the first 2 days following a hysterectomy.

Management of urinary catheters

Urinary bladder catheterization is a standard practice in all types of hysterectomy. A deflated urinary bladder is less likely to be injured during surgery. The indwelling catheter is postoperatively continued to monitor urinary output, detect hematuria which may indicate urinary tract injury, and prevent urinary retention which complicates 10% to 20% of patients during the initial 24 hours of surgery. Urinary catheterization, on the other hand, increases incidence of urinary tract infection and delays ambulation and, thus, should be removed as soon as possible. In general, the indwelling urinary bladder catheter can be removed 12 hours (but not more than 24 hours) after an uncomplicated hysterectomy.

Surgical Complications of Hysterectomy

Hemorrhage

The mean and 90th percentile volume of blood loss during hysterectomy for benign diseases are 100 ml and 400 ml respectively. The risk factors for excessive blood loss are uterine volume of more than 250 ml, pelvic adhesive disease, long operation duration exceeding 3 hours, and gross obesity (BMI >35). Large volume of intraoperative blood loss is associated with higher rates of transfusion of blood and blood products, return to operation, and readmission to hospital.

In the postoperative period, a patient who has a significant ongoing hemorrhage may appear pale and experience lethargy, dizziness, tachycardia, hypotension, or in severe cases, hypovolemic shock. Hourly postoperative monitoring of vital signs and physical inspections are critical during the first 24 hours following hysterectomy. When clinical signs warrant it, a full blood count should be performed to assess the severity of hypohemoglobinemia, although it is the clinical condition of the patient and not the absolute level of hemoglobin that determines the need for blood transfusion.

The cardinal signs indicative of ongoing hemorrhage in a post-operative patient are progressive deterioration of clinical condition and vital signs, as well as increasing abdominal distension or vaginal bleeding. This is a surgical emergency, and it is critical to quickly return to the operating room to secure hemostasis early in the clinical evolution of hemorrhage. In the situation where the patient is in a stable condition, an urgent consultation with an interventional radiologist is needed to determine whether an angiographic investigation and arterial embolization procedure should be carried out.

Surgical Site Infections

The incidence of surgical site infection is approximately 5% and is more common in abdominal hysterectomy than in laparoscopic hysterectomy. Comorbidities carrying high risk of surgical site infection include diabetes mellitus, chronic obstructive airway diseases, being overweight or obesity, American Society of Anesthesiologists class ≥ 3, and chronic smoking. Perioperative blood transfusion and long operating time exceeding 180 minutes are surgical events that increase risk of surgical site infection.

Following hysterectomy, the common sites of surgical wound infection include abdominal wounds, the vaginal vault, pelvic cellulitis, and less commonly abscess formation. They typically present clinically 5 to 7 days after surgery with fever, abdominal or wound pain, wound swelling and discharge, or vaginal bleeding or discharge in cases of vaginal vault cellulitis.

Signs and symptoms of infection

Abdominal wound infection

In the form of wound cellulitis, the overlying skin is erythematous, edematous, warm, and tender. Before a clinical wound abscess develops, a localized or generalized subdermal induration can be elicited on wound palpation. Abscess formation is confirmed by purulent discharge and presence of a fluctuant swelling in the wound.

Vaginal vault cellulitis

Clinical diagnosis is made upon detection of the presence of vaginal discharge and vault tenderness on digital examination. There may be an associated vault hematoma.

Pelvic abscess

This occurs in 1% of cases following hysterectomy. In addition to the general signs and symptoms of inflammation and persistent fever, there may be associated signs of urinary bladder or rectal irritation such as dysuria and frequent micturition, as well as increased urge and frequency of defecation or diarrhea. A tender pelvic mass may be palpable during a bimanual examination.

Investigations of surgical site infection

Microbiological tests

A relevant sample from the wound is taken for laboratory tests to identify the micro-organisms involved and their sensitivity to antibiotics.

The micro-organisms reported in 90% of surgical infections in gynecology comprise gram-positive staphylococcus and streptococcus species, gram-negative bacilli such as E. coli, klebsiella pneumoniae and proteus species, anaerobic gram-positive cocci such as peptoccoci and peptostreptococci species, and anaerobic gram-negative bacilli such as bacteroides and prevotella species.

Blood culture is indicated only if a patient appears ill, is immunocompromised, or is at risk of endocarditis.

Imaging studies

A pelvic ultrasound scan is indicated if vaginal vault hematoma or a pelvic abscess is suspected.

A computerized tomography study of the abdomen and pelvis is useful for investigating suspected cases of intra-abdominal abscess not identified from ultrasound scanning. One should be reminded of the surgical dictum "pus somewhere, pus nowhere, pus under the diaphragm". It also allows for an alternative diagnosis of fever from sepsis to ovarian vein thrombosis.

Management of surgical site infection

Antibiotic therapy

The patient should immediately be treated with a broad-spectrum antibiotic, such as cephazolin or amoxicillin-clavulanic acid, which covers almost 90% of micro-organisms found in such surgical site infections. Oral administration is appropriate for mild cellulitis, but for more severe infections or when an abscess formation is suspected, the antibiotic of choice should be administered intravenously until systemic signs and symptoms of infection have subsided before converting to oral therapy. A good clinical response is usually seen within 48 to 72 hours of commencing antibiotic treatment. In the presence of an abscess, a prolonged period of oral antibiotics is necessary for successful control of the infection.

Drainage of abscess

The standard treatment of wound abscess is by surgical drainage. The infected abdominal wound is laid open for abscess evacuation, debridement, and irrigation. The wound is also left to heal by secondary intention.

A pelvic abscess may be amenable to ultrasound-guided or CT scan-guided insertion of a drain either transvaginally or transcutaneously over the abdomen. In other cases, a laparotomy is needed for complete drainage of the abscess.

Urinary Tract Infection

The incidence of clinical urinary tract infection varies from 5% in abdominal and laparoscopic hysterectomy to 8% in vaginal hysterectomy. The incidence is higher if one includes asymptomatic bacteriuria, which significantly prolongs the duration of hospital stay and the overall cost of hysterectomy.

The risk of urinary tract infection is closely related to the use and duration of indwelling urinary catheterization, age and postmenopausal status of the patient, prior urinary symptoms such as voiding difficulties, and constipation.

Patients with postoperative fever, urinary retention, dysuria, and frequent micturition, hematuria, or abdominal pain should have their midstream urine obtained for bacteriological investigation of potential urinary tract infection. Micro-organisms found in urinary tract infection include both gram-positive and gram-negative bacteria and fungi. The most common culprits are Escherichia coli, Klebsiella pneumoniae, Proteus mirabilis, Enterococcus faecalis, Staphylococcus saprophyticus, and Group-B streptococcus.

The first-line antibacterial therapeutic agents should be based on laboratory evidence of microbial sensitivity to therapeutic agents. When empirical treatment is indicated, the choice of therapeutic agents should be based on microbial sensitivity in the local community.

Intestinal Obstruction

Small bowel obstruction is an uncommon but serious complication of hysterectomy. The incidence of early small bowel obstruction within the first 30 days of hysterectomy for benign diseases is 0.6%, half of which occurs during the first 5 days of the initial hospital admission. The risk factors for small bowel obstruction include using the abdominal route for hysterectomy, previous pelvic or abdominal surgeries, adhesiolysis, intraoperative visceral injuries, and long operating time. Other risk factors include perioperative blood transfusion and sepsis.

The cardinal signs and symptoms of small bowel obstruction are vomiting and abdominal pain. Paralytic ileus presents with a distended abdomen with absence of bowel sounds. In contrast, mechanical small bowel obstruction is characterized by a distended abdomen with increased bowel sounds. A CT scan of the abdomen may demonstrate the level of mechanical obstruction, localization of sepsis, or extravasation of contrast media in visceral or urinary tract injuries.

In the absence of other associated organ injuries, the great majority, or 80%, of small bowel obstruction resolves with nonsurgical management involving gastrointestinal decompression via nasogastric suction, intravenous fluid resuscitation, and treatment of sepsis.

Olgivie's Syndrome, first described by Sir Heneage Ogilvie in 1948, is a rare complication that can occur after, but is not specific to, hysterectomy. Total laparoscopic hysterectomy is not exempt from this complication. The patient experiences increasing abdominal pain and distension as seen in any case of bowel obstruction. Abdominal X-rays reveal a grossly distended ascending colon and caecum in the absence of mechanical obstruction in the colon distally. In untreated cases, the progression of the condition leads to ischemic necrosis and perforation of the caecum, carrying a mortality rate of 5% to 10%. Prompt colonic decompression with colonoscopy and treatment with neostigmine, an anticholinesterase inhibitor, has been shown to be successful in 85% of cases.

Specific Organ Injuries

Ureteric Injury

Urinary tract injuries are well-recognized complications of hysterectomy. They are associated with increased operation time, blood loss and blood transfusion, longer hospital stay, more frequent readmission and reoperation, and various other adverse events overall.

Hysterectomy is the most common cause of iatrogenic ureteric injuries in the pelvis. The overall incidence ranges from 0.5% to 1.5%, being more common in laparoscopic hysterectomy than in abdominal or vaginal hysterectomy. Improvements in laparoscopic surgical technique and surgical experience in recent years have resulted in a decline in the incidence of ureteric injuries, reaching a level similar with other types of hysterectomy. Ironically, a great majority of ureteric injuries in hysterectomy for benign diseases occurs in pelvises with minimal pathology. In a retrospective survey of elective hysterectomy for benign disorders between 2001 and 2010 in the UK, the incidence of ureteric injuries was 0.53% overall — lowest for vaginal hysterectomy and highest for laparoscopic hysterectomy. When grouped by pathology, hysterectomy for endometriosis had the highest incidence of ureteric injury with an occurrence rate of 1 in 60. The individual incidence by types of hysterectomy is shown in the table below:

Crude incidence of ureteric injuries among women who underwent elective hysterectomies for benign gynecological conditions in the UK.			
Types of hysterectomy	**Total number of cases**	**Ureteric injury (cases)**	**Incidence rate (%)**
Laparoscopic	14,692	94	0.64
Vaginal	130,179	159	0.12
Abdominal, total	156,263	719	0.46
Abdominal, subtotal	21,323	108	0.51
Overall	202,457	1080	0.53

Risk factors for ureteric injuries include pathology causing the uterus to be grossly enlarged to beyond 12 weeks in gestational size, ovarian cyst or tumor of 5 cm or more in diameter, endometriosis, pelvic inflammatory disease with adhesions, prior pelvic surgeries, and radiation therapy. Types of ureteric injuries include ligation or kinking by sutures, transection (partial or complete), laceration, and ischemic necrosis from thermal (electrocautery) injuries or damage to the vascular supply of the ureter. Injuries are most commonly seen at the sites of infundibulopelvic ligament near the ovarian fossa, posterior to the uterine artery, and the vaginal angles on closure of the vaginal cuff. The injury may be unilateral, bilateral, or in combination with urinary bladder cystotomy.

Clinical presentations and management

Intraoperative

When a ureteric crushing injury or ligation occurs, the surgical clamp and the suture are immediately removed. The extent and severity of the injury is assessed and ureteric peristalsis is to be observed. An intraoperative urologic consult is called for to achieve optimal management.

When a ureteric transection is suspected, the diagnosis may be confirmed by observing for ureteric extravasation of a dye after intravenous injection of either 10 ml of indigo carmine or methylene blue with 20 mg furosemide. More specifically, a fluoroscopic retrograde uretero–pyelography will detect the location and extent as well as nature of the ureteric injury. Immediate repair will lead to the best surgical outcome. Possible treatment options include expectant management with observation, ureteric stenting, ureteroureterostomy reanastomosis, and ureteroneocystostomy procedures.

Immediate postoperative

Approximately 20% of ureteric injuries following a hysterectomy present during the same hospital admission for the primary surgery. Clinical presentation includes watery vaginal discharge, prolonged ileus, hematuria, inability to pass urine, fever, frank pain, and anuria in cases of bilateral ureteric ligation. The diagnostic procedure depends on clinical presentation.

Watery vaginal discharge: This can be evaluated with a bedside three-swab test to distinguish ureterovaginal fistulas (UVFs) from vesicovaginal fistulas (VVFs) and urinary incontinence. Three surgical swabs are inserted into the vagina apex, mid vagina, and lower vagina. The urinary bladder is filled with 10 ml of methylene blue diluted in 100 ml of water. The patient is asked to walk around for 10 minutes before the vaginal swabs are removed for diagnostic interpretation according to the pattern of soaking and staining. The following table provides a guide for interpreting the three-swab test (VVF = vesicovaginal fistula, UVF = ureterovaginal fistula):

Swab soaking	Blue staining			Interpretation
	Swab at vaginal apex	Swab in mid vagina	Swab in lower vagina	
Yes	Yes or no	Yes	No	VVF
Yes	Yes	No	No	UVF
Yes	No	No	Yes	Urinary incontinence
No	No	No	No	No urinary tract lesions

Increased pelvic drainage output: In cases presenting with a large volume of watery output in a pelvic drain, the possibility of it being urine can be evaluated with creatinine measurement. High fluid content of creatinine confirms the presence of urine.

Loin pain, ileus, and/or anuria: Imaging studies of the urinary tract is the best mode of investigation for both detection and determination for the nature of injury. Intravenous urography (IVU) or a CT urogram can demonstrate the integrity of the urinary tract, site of contrast media extravasation, hydronephrosis and site of obstruction, and renal dysfunction. It is generally believed that IVU is superior to a CT scan in establishing the continuity of the ureter as CT scans only provide cross-sectional images at intervals.

In addition, a comprehensive laboratory evaluation with a full blood count, serum urea and electrolytes, and bacteriological culture and antibiotic sensitivity testing on a midstream urinary specimen are necessary in any suspected cases of urinary tract injury.

Surgical repair techniques are similar to the intraoperative discovery of injury during hysterectomy.

Delayed presentation

Ureteric injuries identified after initial hospitalization for hysterectomy accounted for 80% of all cases. On average, the median time from primary hysterectomy to identification of ureteric injuries is 4 days (between 1.5 to 11 days) for obstruction and 11 days (between 8 to 20 days) for ureterovaginal fistula. The presenting symptoms are mainly continuous vaginal watery discharge, hematuria, dysuria, difficulty in passing urine, and loin or back pain. In some chronic cases such as ureteric stenosis, hydronephrosis and loss of ipsilateral kidney function may present long after the primary surgery.

Approximately 11% of women with reported ureteric injuries end up with ureteric fistulae. The diagnostic techniques are imaging studies with an IVU or CT urogram and serum level of urea, creatinine, and electrolytes. The treatment is mostly conservative with observation or ureteric stenting. Other options similar to those carried out for suspected ureteric injury during the immediate postoperative period are performed in some individual cases.

Urinary Bladder Injury

The incidence of bladder injury associated with hysterectomy is estimated to be 0.8% to 1.5%, or 3 times more common than ureteric injuries. In comparison, vaginal hysterectomy has the lowest incidence of bladder injuries compared to abdominal (relative risk = 1.2) and laparoscopic hysterectomy (relative risk = 3.0). The single most important risk factor, a history of repeated cesarean sections, carries a four-fold increased risk of bladder injury in hysterectomy. Among women with more than two caesarean sections, for example, the rate of unintentional cystotomy has been reported to be 6% for abdominal hysterectomy, 11% for vaginal hysterectomy, and 21% for laparoscopic hysterectomy.

Types of urinary bladder injuries include cystotomy from sharp dissection, laceration from tissue stretching or blunt dissection, devascularization from dissection, ligation or electrocauterization, and placement of intraluminal sutures or staples.

The common sites of bladder injuries are:

i.   Bladder base/trigone area: this occurs during dissection of the bladder away from the uterus and cervix.

ii. Bladder dome: injuries at this site can occur with laceration during laparotomy or with punctures by trocars during laparoscopy. The trocar injuries may involve entry and exit punctures.

Presentation of urinary bladder injury

Intraoperative signs

- Bleeding from the muscle layer of the bladder
- Formation of hematoma in the muscle layer of the bladder
- Spillage of urine
- Appearance of catheter balloon
- Routine intraoperative cystoscopic findings: Some unsuspected bladder injuries are discovered in routine intraoperative cystoscopy during hysterectomy. Cystoscopy, however, has a significant false positive and false negative rate in detecting these injuries. The cost effectiveness of universal intraoperative hysterectomy cystoscopy during hysterectpmy during hysterectomy remains unproven.

Intraoperative management

- Intraoperative urological consultation and referral are standard procedures of care.
- Cystotomy: Obvious cases do not require any specific diagnostic test. However, examination of the ureteric orifices is important to ascertain the integrity of the ureters. Cystotomy is repaired by primary closure. The integrity of the bladder is tested with intravesicular distillation of methylene blue solution.

    Free drainage of the bladder with an indwelling urinary catheter for 14 days and prophylactic antibiotics are recommended.
- Partial laceration: The muscular defect is closed with 3/O absorbable sutures and reinforced with overlying peritoneum. The integrity of the bladder is tested with intravesicular distillation of methylene blue solution.
- Hematoma: Conservative management with observation only.

Postoperative signs and symptoms

- Difficulty in passing urine
- Leaking of urine
- Hematuria
- Symptoms of cystitis such as frequent micturition and dysuria
- Urine ascites: Free urine in the peritoneal cavity presenting with abdominal distension and pain.

The most significant sequelae of bladder injuries is the development of VVF, which affects 8% of women with reported bladder injury. The mean time from hysterectomy to detection of VVF is 12.5 days (ranging from 4.8 to 22.3 days).

Preliminary evaluation

- Three-swab test
- Midstream urine for bacteriological investigation
- Serum level of urea, creatinine, and electrolytes

Specific investigations

- Urological referral and consultation: This should be promptly initiated when the three-swab test is positive or in cases where a definitive diagnosis of persistent leaking of urine is uncertain.
- IVU and retrograde cytourethrography to evaluate the integrity of the urinary tract and diagnosis of VVF.
- Cystoscopy: This will confirm the number, size, site, and type of bladder injury.

Management of vesicovaginal fistula

Almost 90% of VVFs after hysterectomy are less than 2 cm in size and located in the supratrigonal part of the posterior bladder wall, incorporated in the vaginal vault scar, or near the vault scar at the anterior vaginal wall.

- Conservative management: Nonsurgical management with prolonged period of urinary bladder catheterization is a possible method of treating a small fistula of less than 1 cm in size. The reported success rate, however, is less than 10%.
- Surgical closure of the fistula: This is the mainstay of treatment of post-hysterectomy VVFs with a success rate of more than 95%, regardless of time of repair within or beyond 12 weeks of the hysterectomy.

  The surgical principle of fistula repair is to achieve watertight closure of the vesical defect without any tension in the wound. In general, gynecologists prefer a vaginal approach with lesser morbidity. This is closely followed, in frequency, by the abdominal approach. More recently, the feasibility of repairs through laparoscopic and robotic approaches have been established.

  The method of VVF repair most favored by gynecologists involves a colpocleisis without excision of the fistula tract was described by Dr William Latzko from New York in 1942. The technique, in brief, includes the following steps:

- With the patient in the lithotomy position, a size-16 Foley catheter is inserted into the bladder lumen through the fistulous opening and the balloon is inflated.
- The fistula is drawn downwards and a circumferential incision is made at a distance of 2 cm from the fistulous opening. This will effectively remove the epithelium of the anterior and posterior vaginal wall around the fistula.
- The anterior and posterior vaginal wall are now approximated by interrupted absorbable sutures (e.g., 0/Vicryl or Monocril sutures) without placing any sutures within the bladder.
- The Foley catheter is removed and the vaginal mucosa is closed. Water tightness is confirmed with bladder instillation of methylene blue or saline.
- Free drainage of the bladder through a transurethral Foley catheter is maintained for 14 days and removed only after a normal cystogram.

Intestinal Injury

Bowel injury is a well-acknowledged risk of hysterectomy. It carries significant mortality and morbidity alongside an increase in operation time, blood loss and blood transfusion, postoperative infection complications, duration of hospital stay, and incidence of readmission. Delay in diagnosis carries a mortality rate as high as 20%.

The overall incidence of bowel injuries in hysterectomy for benign disorders is estimated to be 0.4%. The significant risk factors for bowel injuries are shown in the following table:

Risk factors for intestinal injuries in hysterectomy.

Risk factor	Incidence rate (%)	Odds ratio
Surgical approach		
Vaginal	0.10	1
Laparoscopic	0.20	2.03
Abdominal	1.05	10.49
Adhesiolysis		
No	0.38	1
Yes	1.16	3.45
Type of pathology		
Genital prolapse	0.18	1
Menstrual disorders	0.20	1.10
Uterine fibroids	0.47	2.68
Endometriosis	0.59	3.35

Most bowel injuries are detected and repaired during primary surgery of hysterectomy. However, in laparoscopic hysterectomy, almost up to 40% of bowel injuries are diagnosed in the postoperative period. This is partly because injuries caused by a Veress needle during creation of pneumoperitoneum may be undetectable, and some thermal injuries may be a distance away from the site of surgery and are unrecognizable at the time of surgery.

The mean time for postoperative diagnosis of bowel injuries is 3 days. The main presenting signs and symptoms are:

- Peritonitis
- Abdominal pain
- Ileus
- Fever and leukocytosis
- Abdominal distension
- Rectovaginal fistula
- Abdominal abscess
- Septic shock
- Acute respiratory distress syndrome

Diagnosis of bowel injuries is based on clinical history of risk factors and surgical encounters, as well as clinical examination of the patient's condition. A CT scan may provide evidence of intra-abdominal abscesses.

Management of bowel injuries include:

- Intravenous fluid resuscitation and blood transfusion when indicated;
- Intravenous antibiotics to cover intestinal flora;
- Laboratory evaluations: Full blood count, urea, and electrolytes;
- Prompt laparotomy with peritoneal larvage and examination of the entire gastrointestinal tract for injuries;
- Delayed diagnosis often results in severe infection of the injured part that calls for bowel resection and reanastomosis;
- Inserting a large peritoneal drainage before abdominal closure.

Venous Thromboembolism (VTE)

VTE, which involves either deep vein thrombosis (DVT), pulmonary embolism (PE), or both, occurs at an estimated rate of 0.2% following hysterectomy for benign conditions. The risk is lowest (0.1%) in vaginal hysterectomy and laparoscopic hysterectomy and

2.5 times higher in abdominal hysterectomy. Despite being an uncommon occurrence, pulmonary embolism is the most common cause of mortality for hysterectomy for benign conditions.

Most cases of DVT are asymptomatic. Incidence of pulmonary embolism as high as 40% has been reported from research on women with DVT. Many of these women with pulmonary embolism had little or no clinical symptoms. On the other hand, patients may present with severe symptoms of pulmonary embolism — even fatality — without prior diagnosis of DVT. The great majority of cases of thromboembolism following hysterectomy presents only days after discharge from hospital and are never known to gynecologists. The role of good perioperative care lies in identifying women with high risk of thromboembolism and taking appropriate preventive measures.

Risk Factors for Venous Thromboembolism

There are several well-recognized constitutional and medical conditions that raise the risk of VTE in patients. These conditions allow for objective stratification of risk of VTE for individual patients.

One example of risk scoring that can be adapted for clinical practice is provided below:

Point	Each condition scores individually (Caprini score)
1	41–60 years of age, BMI >25, cigarette smoking, swollen legs, varicose veins, combined oral contraceptive pill use, myocardial infarctions, congestive cardiac failure, sepsis within 1 month
2	61–74 years of age, bedrest >72 hours
3	≥75 years of age, inherited clotting factors, SLE/APS
5	Stroke within 1 month

*Modified from Bahl V, Hu HM, Henke PK, Wakefield TW, Campbell DA Jr, Caprini JA. A validation study of a retrospective venous thromboembolism risk scoring method. *Ann Surg.* Feb 2010;251(2):344–50.

Methods of Venous Thromboembolism Prophylaxis

Graduated compression stockings (elastic stockings)

Venous flow in the lower limbs is improved by graduated compression stockings. Its perioperative use has been shown to reduce the incidence of VTE in surgical patients by 65%. It is low cost and safe, except for potential skin complications such as blistering and ulceration. Knee-length stockings are preferred to the full-lenth lower limb stockings.

Intermittent pneumatic compression devices

Continual use of intermittent pneumatic compression (IPC) devices from the time of surgery until the patient is fully ambulatory and ready for hospital discharge has been shown to reduce the risk of both asymptomatic and distal DVT by 60%, which is as effective as low molecular weight heparin and low-dose heparin.

Low molecular weight heparin

Low molecular weight heparin (LMWH) has been shown to be as effective as unfractionated low-dose heparin in reducing the risk of VTE among high-risk surgical patients. The benefits and risks of these pharmacological agents in hysterectomy for benign conditions remain controversial. The table below outlines the estimated harms and benefits of these agents.

Benefits		Harms	
Type of VTE	Case reduction per 1,000 patients	Type of harm	Case increase per 1,000 patients
Mortality	4	Major bleeding	6
Symptomatic PE	2	Reoperation	0
Proximal DVT	4		
Distal DVT	0		

The suggested best contemporary practices for perioperative VTE prophylaxis for hysterectomy for benign conditions include:

Risk grouping	Cumulative Caprini score	Presumed incidence of VTE (%)	Prophylactic measures	
			Stockings or IPC	LMWH (if not at high risk of bleeding)
Low	2 or less	0.1 to 1.5	Yes	No
Moderate	3 to 4	3	Yes	Yes
High	5 or more	6	Yes	Yes

The lack of consensus on VTE prophylaxis is due to the limited data available on the efficacy and cost effectiveness of specific interventions for risk reduction of VTE for hysterectomy for benign conditions.

Preparing Patients for Discharge

Patients undergoing an uncomplicated hysterectomy for benign conditions typically stay in hospital for one to four days, depending on whether the vaginal, laparoscopic, or abdominal surgical approach is used. The purpose of hospital stay is to detect and treat any immediate surgical adverse events and achieve optimal surgical pain control. A large part of the process of recovery from surgery takes place at home.

Discharge Criteria

Before discharge, the surgeon must be confident that the patient has no immediate adverse surgical events and is at low risk for such events during the ensuing convalescence period of 30 days. The important observations to establish confidence include:

1. Normal vital signs
2. No excessive vaginal bleeding or watery discharge
3. Satisfactory condition of surgical wounds
4. Satisfactory surgical pain control
5. Adequate independent ambulatory activity
6. Satisfactory oral diet intake
7. Satisfactory voluntary excretory functions

The same parameters also help patients to be confident to leave the hospital and manage their convalescence on their own.

Patient Education

Adequate patient education not only improves the confidence of patients and reduces unnecessary clinic attendance, but also improves surgical outcomes by empowering patients to look out for abnormal recovering processes and prompt early remedial intervention. This is an important process to improve the overall experience of patients in the journey of hysterectomy.

Expected physiological changes

As some symptoms of physiological changes following major surgery are unfamiliar and worrisome to patients, the most common changes should be adequately explained to them.

Surgery-related changes

Abdominal and wound pain are expected following surgery. In uncomplicated cases, the pain should ease steadily day-by-day and become minimal or completely disappear by the end of the first week of surgery. It is recommended that patients continue with regular analgesics established during their hospital stay.

It is normal to experience an exacerbation of pain momentarily during physical exertion on the abdomen.

Swollen abdominal wounds: Abdominal wounds may appear a little swollen and feel lumpy when pressed gently with the fingers. Skin adjacent to the wound may also feel numb on touching.

Vaginal bleeding: Unfamiliar to women, hysterectomy carries a surgical wound at the vaginal vault. Light vaginal bleeding may continue for up to two weeks but in reducing quantity over time.

Urethral soreness: After removal of the urinary catheter, there may be experience of soreness in the urethra on passing urine during the first few days following hysterectomy.

Constipation: Retarded bowel motility resulting in clinical constipation is common after hysterectomy. This change is brought about by a number of intraoperative and perioperative factors, including the use of certain medications, particularly opioid and opioid-like analgesia and some anesthetic agents, the surgical process and associated inflammatory reactions, intraoperative manipulation of bowels, and changes in dietary habits during hospital stay and early phases of convalescence.

Catabolism-related changes

The human body undergoes a state of catabolism in response to the stress of any major surgery. This is characterized biochemically by deranged glucose metabolism, insulin resistance, increased protein breakdown, and negative nitrogen balance. The degree of catabolic changes is directly proportional to the extent of surgery and associated inflammatory reactions, use of certain neuraxial anesthetic agents and opioid and opioid-like analgesia, and the patient's nutritional state.

List of Clinical Symptoms of Catabolic Metabolism After Hysterectomy:

- Fatigue
- General weakness
- Shortness of breaths
- Dizziness
- Weight loss

Postsurgical catabolic metabolism may take several weeks to recover. Both the severity and duration of clinical presentation (table) of the catabolic state vary widely between individual patients.

Ovarian hormone-related changes

When a premenopausal woman has both ovaries removed at the time of hysterectomy, she enters an immediate state of menopausal estrogen and progesterone deficiency, also known as surgical menopause. Additionally, there is loss of the ovarian source of androgens. The symptoms of these hormonal deficiencies are summarized in the following table:

Possible symptoms of surgical menopause in the absence of estrogen replacement therapy:

Time lapse since surgical menopause	Type of symptoms
Immediate or soon	Hot flushes, night sweats
	Vaginal dryness
	Reduced sex drive (libido)
	Loss of fertility
	Mood and cognitive changes
	Increased rate of bone loss
Late	Increased risk of osteoporosis and fractures
	Increased risk of cardiovascular diseases
Life-time risk	Increased overall mortality rate
	Increased risk of Alzheimer's disease

The onset and severity of clinical symptoms (table) from the time of surgery show great variation between individual women, being more obvious and more significant in younger women or those below 45 years old.

These symptoms are induced by estrogen deficiency and are responsive to estrogen replacement therapy. Almost 90% of hot flushes and increased perspiration resolves on estrogen replacement therapy. Reduced libido, on the other hand, is related to testosterone deficiency and the woman may elect to undergo testosterone replacement therapy. The decision on the initiation of estrogen and testosterone replacement therapy is a combined decision between the gynecologist and the patient.

Actionable Pathological Conditions

Discharge from hospital during the early stage of surgical recovery is safe only if women are instructed on some signs and symptoms of late complications of surgery. Early recognition and medical intervention are important for optimal treatment outcomes.

Secondary hemorrhage

Onset of vaginal bleeding after initial days of absence or little bleeding are seen in up to 2% of all hysterectomies. Many of these cases are reactionary bleeding associated with increased physical activities or exertion, including sexual intercourse. The bleeding is generally light and settles on resting.

Pathological secondary hemorrhage, which occurs more rarely at around 0.1% to 1%, carries potentially grave consequences. The mean interval between hysterectomy and onset of secondary hemorrhage is 10 days, and the range extends from 3 to 21 days. It is most often caused by an ascending infection of the vaginal vault by anogenital bacteria. Bleeding can also result from a vaginal vault hematoma, bleeding vessels, laceration in the vaginal vault, or vault dehiscence.

Patients should be instructed on actions to take upon seeing vaginal bleeding during the recovery period. If the bleeding is not more than a normal menstrual flow, she should observe whether the bleeding stops after a period of rest from physical activities. A persistently moderate amount of vaginal bleeding should prompt her to visit her family doctor for a definitive diagnosis and initiation of appropriate antibiotic therapy.

Any vaginal bleeding in excess of her prior experience of the day of heavy menstruation flow should prompt her to seek immediate attention from an emergency medical service for comprehensive evaluation and treatment. Delays in instituting medical therapy may put the patient in a desperate state of cardiovascular compromise.

Surgical site infection

Surgical site infection after hysterectomy occurs from infection of surgical incisional wounds, the vaginal vault, or the pelvis within 30 days of surgery. Infection of the incisional site can be superficial or deep, and pelvic infection includes pelvic cellulitis and abscess. The clinical presentation is a combination of signs and symptoms including:

— Abdominal pain or tenderness
— Wound pain or tenderness
— Wound swelling
— Wound redness
— Wound heat

— Spontaneous wound dehiscence
— Fever (>38°C)
— Vaginal discharge with a foul odor
— Purulent drainage from the wound, vagina, or pelvic drainage tube

Surgical site infection is the second most common indication for readmission to hospital. The risk factors for infection include old age, diabetes mellitus, a high BMI of >30, cigarette smoking, and perioperative blood transfusion.

Urinary tract infection

Symptomatic lower genital tract infection occurs in 5% of hysterectomy and presents with frequent micturition, dysuria, hematuria, or suprapubic abdominal pain.

Venous thromboembolism

Signs and symptoms of VTE should be made known to patients for prompt medical attention:

— Swollen leg
— Leg pain when weight is put on it or during walking
— Tender leg
— Warmness in the leg
— Shortness of breaths
— Chest pain on deep breathing

Measures to Enhance Recovery

Nutrition

A healthy balanced diet with adequate calorie intake provides the necessary daily nutritional physiological requirement. There is no evidence that adjustment in dietary composition or supplementation of micronutritional elements in megadoses alters the course of surgery associated with catabolic metabolism.

A balanced diet and adequate hydration play an important role in preventing constipation and urinary tract infection.

Patients should stop cigarette smoking, while alcohol consumption should be kept to none or within the recommended quantity of responsible social drinking.

Physical exercise

Physical exercise not involving the sites of surgery does not hamper wound recovery. On the contrary, it may reduce loss of muscle mass associated with bed rest and, thus, improve the general well-being of the patient.

Patients are encouraged to begin low intensity physical exercise as soon as they can begin ambulating after hysterectomy. The intensity of exercise is increased incrementally to the presurgery state by the end of four to six weeks.

Return to Normal Personal and Vocational Activity

Daily chores

Light intensity daily chores can be resumed after hospital discharge.

Car driving

Anesthetic medications and some analgesics are sedatives, which have a negative impact on psychomotor functions. One should not drive a motor vehicle until 24 hours or longer after these medications have been ceased.

Sexual intercourse

Patients who do not encounter any complications during recovery can resume sexual intercourse at 6 weeks after hysterectomy, a duration that would have allowed for complete healing of the vaginal vault.

Return to work

Depending on the physical demands of work and the type of hysterectomy, women generally resume full-time work four to six weeks after surgery. Women who have had an abdominal hysterectomy are recommended to begin their vocational work part-time initially and increase their working hours according to their physical condition.

References

ACOG Committee on Gynecologic Practice. (2018) Perioperative pathways: Enhanced recovery after surgery. *Obstet Gynecol* **132**: e120–e130.

Bindu B, Rath G. (2017) Temperature management under general anesthesia: Compulsion or option. *J Anaesthesiol Clin Pharmacol* **33**(3): 306–316.

Black JD, de Haydu C, Fan L, *et al.* (2014) Surgical site infections in gynecology. *Obstet Gynecol Surv* **69**(8): 501–510. doi: 10.1097/OGX.0000000000000102. PMID: 25144613.

Brummer THI, Jalkanen J, Fraser J, *et al.* (2011) FINHYST, a prospective study of 5279 hysterectomies: Complications and their risk factors. *Hum Reprod* **26**: 1741–1751.

Kahr HS, Thorlacius-Ussing O, Christiansen OB, *et al.* (2017) Venous thromboembolic complications to hysterectomy for benign disease: A nationwide cohort study. *JMIG* **25**(4): 715–723. https://doi.org/10.1016/j.jmig.2017.11.017

Kiran A, Hilton P, Cromwell DA. (2016) The risk of ureteric injury associated with hysterectomy: A 10-year retrospective cohort study. *BJOG* **123**: 1184–1191.

Lethaby A, Vollenhoven B, Sowter M. (2002) Efficacy of pre-operative gonadotrophin hormone releasing analogues for women with uterine fibroids undergoing hysterectomy or myomectomy: A systematic review. *BJOG* **109**: 1097–1108.

Lirk P, Thiry J, Bonnet M-P, *et al.* (2019) Pain management after laparoscopic hysterectomy: Systematic review of literature and PROSPECT recommendations. *Reg Anesth Pain Med* **44**: 425–436.

Maresh MJ, Metcalfe MA, McPherson K, *et al.* (2002) The VALUE national hysterectomy study: Description of the patients and their surgery. *BJOG* **109**(3): 302–312. doi: 10.1111/j.1471-0528.2002.01282.x.

Perniola A, Fant F, Magnuson A, *et al.* (2014) Postoperative pain after abdominal hysterectomy: A randomized, double-blind, controlled trial comparing continuous infusion vs patient-controlled intraperitoneal injection of local anesthetic. *Br J Anaesth* **112**: 328–336.

RCOG Scientific Paper. Enhanced recovery in gynecology.

RCOG Scientific Impact Paper No. 36 February 2013.

Schricker T, Lattermann R. (2015) Perioperative catabolism. *Can Anesth* **62**: 182–193.

Sheyn D, Bretschneider E, Mahajan ST, *et al.* (2019) Incidence and risk factors of early postoperative small bowel obstruction in patients undergoing hysterectomy for benign indications. *Am J Obstet Gynecol* **220**: 251.e1–e9.

Swenson CW, Berger MB, Kamdar NS, *et al.* (2015) Risk factors for venous thromboembolism after hysterectomy. *Obstet Gynecol* **125**(5): 1139–1144.

Appendix

Table showing the number of cases of laparotomy, laparoscopy, and vaginal hysterectomy performed by the author between 1997 and 2017 in a single institution:

Types of surgery	Number of cases
Laparotomy	**2,939**
• Total hysterectomy with bilateral salpingectomy	340
• Total hysterectomy with unilateral or bilateral salpingo-oophorectomy	634
• Total hysterectomy with pelvic lymphadenectomy	135
• Total hysterectomy, omentectomy, and pelvic lymphadenectomy	446
• Wertheim hysterectomy with pelvic lymphadenectomy	129
• Myomectomy	352
• Salpingo-oophorectomy, unilateral or bilateral	126
• Ovarian cystectomy, unilateral or bilateral	171
• Salpingectomy, unilateral or bilateral	12
• Lower segment cesarean section	394
• Others	200
Laparoscopy	**1,445**
• Total hysterectomy	81
• Total hysterectomy with unilateral or bilateral salpingo-oophorectomy	97
• Total hysterectomy with pelvic lymphadenectomy	93
• Myomectomy	15

(Continued)

(Continued)

Types of surgery	Number of cases
• Salpingo-oophorectomy, unilateral or bilateral	92
• Salpingectomy, unilateral or bilateral	536
• Salpingotomy, unilateral or bilateral	35
• Tubal sterilization	68
• Hydrotubation	168
• Others	260
Vaginal hysterectomy	**342**
• Vaginal hysterectomy	193
• Vaginal hysterectomy with bilateral salpingectomy	9
• Vaginal hysterectomy with unilateral or bilateral salpingo-oophorectomy	57
• Vaginal hysterectomy with pelvic floor repairs	83

Index